The Syringe Driver

Oxford University Press makes no representation, express or implied, that the drug dosages in this book are correct. Readers must therefore always check the product information and clinical procedures with the most up to date published product information and data sheets provided by the manufacturers and the most recent codes of conduct and safety regulations. The authors and the publishers do not accept responsibility or legal liability for any errors in the text or for the misuse or misapplication of material in this work.

The Syringe Driver
Continuous subcutaneous infusions in palliative care
Second edition

Andrew Dickman
Specialist Principal Pharmacist, Palliative Care Team,
Whiston Hospital, Prescot, Merseyside, UK

Jennifer Schneider
Senior Lecturer in Pharmacy,
University of Newcastle, Newcastle, UK

James Varga
Palliative Care Pharmacist,
Pain and Palliative Care Association, Florida, USA

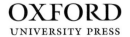
OXFORD
UNIVERSITY PRESS

OXFORD
UNIVERSITY PRESS

Great Clarendon Street, Oxford OX2 6DP

Oxford University Press is a department of the University of Oxford.
It furthers the University's objective of excellence in research, scholarship,
and education by publishing worldwide in

Oxford New York

Auckland Cape Town Dar es Salaam Hong Kong Karachi Kuala Lumpur Madrid
Melbourne Mexico City Nairobi New Delhi Taipei Tokyo Shanghai

With offices in

Argentina Austria Brazil Chile Czech Republic France Greece Guatemala Hungary
Italy Japan South Korea Poland Portugal Singapore Switzerland Thailand Turkey
Ukraine Vietnam

Published in the United States
by Oxford University Press Inc., New York

© Dickman, Schneider, and Varga 2005

First edition published 2002

This edition published 2005

A catalogue record for this title is available from the British Library

Library of Congress Cataloging in Publication Data
(Data available)

ISBN 0 19 856693 X (Pbk)

10 9 8 7 6 5 4 3 2 1

Typeset by Cepha Imaging Pvt. Ltd., Bangalore, India
Printed in Great Britain
on acid-free paper by
Ashford Colour Press Ltd, Gosport, Hampshire

Preface

The syringe driver is a simple and cost-effective method of delivering a continuous subcutaneous infusion (CSCI). A CSCI provides a safe and effective way of drug administration and can be used to maintain symptom control in patients who are no longer able to take oral medication.

There have been several developments in this field since the first edition, including new devices and drugs; these changes have been incorporated into this edition. There is also a wealth of stability data provided, covering an extensive list of drug combinations.

This book serves as a valuable reference source, providing extensive information pertaining to the use of CSCIs. The first chapter provides an in depth overview of syringe drivers and CSCIs, including detailed setup information. The second chapter provides revised and referenced information relating to most drugs likely to be administered via a CSCI using a syringe driver. Drugs that should only be used by, or on the recommendation of, a specialist palliative care centre are clearly marked. The third chapter provides information relating to the control of specific symptoms that are often encountered when CSCIs are required. The fourth and final chapter contains an extensive, referenced (where possible) list of physical and chemical stability data relating to drug combinations used for subcutaneous administration.

Important note

Physical stability data comes from two sources in this book—the laboratory and the clinical setting. Mixtures within this book are termed physically compatible if they remained colourless, clear, and free from particulate matter over the specified time; additionally, for clinical data, the expected outcome was realized.

References to chemical stability, where available, will be found in Chapter 2 under each drug monograph and tabulated in Chapter 4 if the data are available.

Finally, stability data mentioned here can only serve as an indicator and may not apply to all situations.

All information included in this book is correct at the time of writing. The majority of drugs mentioned in this book do not have product licences for administration via CSCI (i.e. their use is 'off label'). Practitioners are advised to check local information with their respective regulatory body. Whilst every effort has been made to ensure accuracy, responsibility remains with the prescriber. Neither the authors nor the publisher can accept responsibility for any errors or omissions that may be made.

Andrew Dickman
Jennifer Schneider
James Varga
2004

Contents

Abbreviations

General

AUS	Australia
LCD	Liquid crystal display
PVC	Polyvinyl chloride
UK	United Kingdom
USA	United States of America
UV	Ultraviolet (light)
WHO	World Health Organization

Medical

5-HT_2	5-Hydroxytriptamine (serotonin) type 2 (receptor)
5-HT3	5-Hydroxytriptamine (serotonin) type 3 (receptor)
$\alpha 2$	Alpha adrenergic type 2 (receptor)
δ	Delta opioid (receptor)
κ	Kappa opioid (receptor)
μ	Mu opioid (receptor)
D_2	Dopamine type 2 (receptor)
H_1	Histamine type 1 (receptor)
CNS	Central nervous system
CSCI(s)	Continuous subcutaneous infusion(s)
CTZ	Chemoreceptor trigger zone
DEX	Dextrose 5% in water
IM	Intramuscular
IV	Intravenous
m/r	Modified release
M3G	Morphine-3-glucuronide
M6G	Morphine-6-glucuronide
NaCl	Sodium chloride 0.9%
NMDA	N-methyl-D-aspartate
NSAID(s)	Non-steroidal anti-inflammatory drug(s)
PO	Orally (*per os*—by mouth)

PRN	When required (*pro re nata*)
SC	Subcutaneously
Stat	Immediately
WFI	Water for Injections

Units

h	Hour(s)
mg	Milligram(s)
ml	Millilitre(s)
mm	Millimetre(s)
s	Seconds(s)
V	Volt(s)

Chapter 1

Continuous subcutaneous infusions and syringe drivers

Introduction

A continuous subcutaneous infusion (CSCI) is an effective method of drug administration that is particularly suited to palliative care. Administration via the oral route should be maintained for as long as practical, although a given patient's condition is likely to deteriorate such that it is no longer possible to administer drugs this way. In such circumstances, (and where possible) the use of a CSCI, via syringe driver, is the preferred method of drug administration to maintain symptom control; rectal administration is not always practical, or acceptable; intravenous injections or infusions should be avoided, particularly as CSCIs are less invasive and as effective; intramuscular administration would be painful, especially if the patient is cachectic.

The use of a CSCI is often wrongly associated with imminent death, not just by the patient or carer, but by health care professionals as well. It should be understood that the use of a syringe driver could be for a multitude of reasons that do not always mean that the end of life is approaching; for example, a CSCI can be employed to control the symptoms of intractable nausea and vomiting.

A syringe driver is generally described as a portable battery-operated device that can be used to deliver a CSCI. Such devices have been available since 1978 when they were introduced for the delivery of desferrioxamine in thalassaemia.[1] They were soon to be used for the administration of drugs to palliative care patients.[2]

A survey in 1992[3] showed that the two most commonly used syringe drivers in several hospices within the UK were the Graseby devices, the MS16A and the MS26 (see Fig. 1.1). In the US, a report showed that approximately 75% of hospices utilized CSCIs.[4] These tended to be larger organizations; there are several factors why this could be so, including an ability to absorb the increased cost over other routes of administration. However, a majority of hospices that utilized CSCIs, employed a cartridge device, as opposed to a syringe driver. The syringe driver has clear cost benefits over cartridge systems. Advances in technology, without a substantial increase in cost, have improved the appeal of the syringe driver as a safe and effective way of delivering a CSCI.

There are currently several syringe drivers available and a new device is currently under development (see Fig. 1.1). The main difference

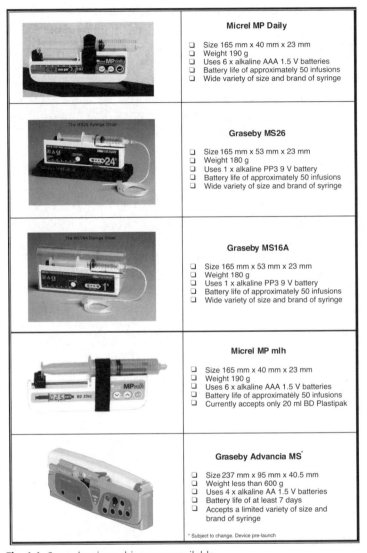

Micrel MP Daily

❏ Size 165 mm x 40 mm x 23 mm
❏ Weight 190 g
❏ Uses 6 x alkaline AAA 1.5 V batteries
❏ Battery life of approximately 50 infusions
❏ Wide variety of size and brand of syringe

Graseby MS26

❏ Size 165 mm x 53 mm x 23 mm
❏ Weight 180 g
❏ Uses 1 x alkaline PP3 9 V battery
❏ Battery life of approximately 50 infusions
❏ Wide variety of size and brand of syringe

Graseby MS16A

❏ Size 165 mm x 53 mm x 23 mm
❏ Weight 180 g
❏ Uses 1 x alkaline PP3 9 V battery
❏ Battery life of approximately 50 infusions
❏ Wide variety of size and brand of syringe

Micrel MP mlh

❏ Size 165 mm x 40 mm x 23 mm
❏ Weight 190 g
❏ Uses 6 x alkaline AAA 1.5 V batteries
❏ Battery life of approximately 50 infusions
❏ Currently accepts only 20 ml BD Plastipak

Graseby Advancia MS*

❏ Size 237 mm x 95 mm x 40.5 mm
❏ Weight less than 600 g
❏ Uses 4 x alkaline AA 1.5 V batteries
❏ Battery life of at least 7 days
❏ Accepts a limited variety of size and brand of syringe

* Subject to change. Device pre-launch

Fig. 1.1 Several syringe drivers are available.

between these devices relates to the rate of delivery. The Graseby MS26 and Micrel MP Daily are arguably the simplest to use and are therefore suggested for use in the palliative care setting. The rate of delivery of these two devices is based on length (mm) per 24 hours. Future legislation may insist that syringe drivers deliver at a rate determined by volume (ml) per unit time (i.e. per hour or 24 hours) rather than length. Accordingly, two additional syringe drivers, Graseby Advancia MS and Micrel MP mlh, are briefly mentioned below.

Indications

There are two popular myths surrounding the use of CSCIs: impending death and superior analgesia. Contrary to these beliefs, a CSCI can be used in a variety of situations (not necessarily implying that death is imminent), and a CSCI should **not** be considered the 'fourth step' of the WHO analgesic ladder; intractable pain is not an indication. See Table 1.1 for accepted indications for use of a CSCI.

Table 1.1 Indications for a continuous subcutaneous infusion

Current route	Indication for CSCI
Oral	Nausea and vomiting
	Dysphagia
	Severe weakness
	Patient request (e.g. a large number of tablets)
Rectal	Diarrhoea
	Bowel obstruction
	Patient preference (particularly the British)
Parenteral	Cachexia
	Fear
	Discomfort
	Infection

Syringe drivers

Important note Mobile phones should not be placed near syringe drivers. All devices described here are designed to fail safe, should high levels of electronomagnetic interference be encountered.

(A) Graseby MS26 and MS16A

These devices are simple to use but are very similar in appearance and fatal errors, due to incorrect identification, continue to be reported.[5] Although the devices are coloured differently, and are clearly labelled on the front, the most commonly encountered issue with these devices relates to confusion between model and delivery rates. The flow rate is determined in the same way on both devices, that is, in mm of syringe travel (MS16A delivers at a rate of mm/hour; MS26 delivers at a rate of mm/24 hours); it is the length of liquid within the syringe, not the volume, which determines the rate of delivery with these syringe drivers. The MS26 and MS16A can deliver a maximum syringe barrel length of 60mm per infusion (this represents the maximum distance that the syringe plunger can be extended and still fit on the device). This allows for greater flexibility in the choice of syringe (brand and size). Note that only Luer Lok™ syringes should be used. Syringes of varying sizes can be attached to these syringe drivers with 35 ml being the largest. With this syringe size, a length of 60 mm equates to approximately 25 ml. Hence, the largest volume of liquid that can be infused is approximately 25 ml. This is important when considering large doses of certain drugs, for example, glycopyrronium (200 mg/ml), midazolam (10 mg/2 ml) or oxycodone (10 mg/ml).

The Differences

The main important difference between these syringe drivers is that the MS26 delivers at a rate set in **mm per 24 hours,** whereas the MS16A delivers at a rate set in **mm per hour.**
Note that delivery is based on the length of liquid and not its volume.

A recent evaluation by the Medicines and Healthcare products Regulatory Authority (MHRA)[5] stated that these two devices are devoid of safety features that would be expected from current technology. The alarms that are available are rudimentary: occlusion (poor response, with a long time to alarm), end of syringe and boost button (see setup below). If the syringe is not fitted correctly, or is tampered with, there will be no alarm, the devices will continue to

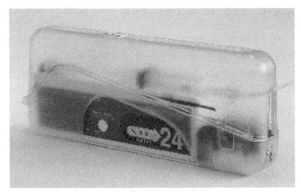

Fig. 1.2 Lockbox for the MS drivers.

work and siphoning may occur. Accidental syringe displacement can be prevented by use of the plastic cover (see Fig. 1.1) and Graseby has recently developed a security device for these drivers in order to prevent tampering (see Fig. 1.2). In the UK, however, such a device has not previously been thought necessary.

The MS26 has a boost button. The use of this is not recommended for several reasons:

◆ There is no lock-out period. Once the boost button is depressed, the device delivers eight boosts and an alarm will sound. The infusion continues. If the button is released and depressed again, a further eight boosts can be delivered, and so on. Hence, there is a potential risk of the whole syringe being delivered this way.

◆ The dose of analgesic delivered by the boost, in relation to the recommended rescue dose for breakthrough pain, is wholly inadequate. For example, consider a syringe with 75 mg diamorphine in 18 ml. A correct rescue dose for breakthrough pain would be 10–15 mg. One boost would deliver less than 1 mg, depending upon the dimensions of the syringe.

◆ Drugs other than analgesics are usually present and boost doses of these should not be given.

◆ The delivery of a boost dose can cause pain at the injection site.

◆ The overall duration of the infusion is reduced, causing problems with renewal.

Important note A 20 ml syringe is the **recommended minimum** for several reasons. Diluting the mixture to the maximum volume may reduce both the risk of adverse site reactions and incompatibility. In addition, the amount of drug wasted in the infusion set will be reduced, so the issue of priming the line becomes less important.

Assembly

1 Fill the syringe with the prescribed drug(s) and dilute the contents up to a maximum length of 60 mm. Use the millimetre scale on the driver for reference.

2 Prime the infusion line, if required (see Box 1.1).

3 Measure the length of barrel against the millimetre scale on the syringe driver, as shown in Fig. 1.3.

4 Set the delivery rate by adjusting the screws on the front of the syringe driver. The rate is derived by dividing the length of the liquid by the required infusion time (in days i.e. 1 for MS26; in hours i.e. 24 for MS16A).

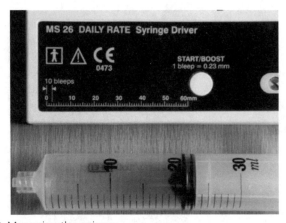

Fig. 1.3 Measuring the syringe.

Box 1.1 The effects of priming the line

If the syringe is measured *before* priming the infusion line, the infusion will finish early:

$$\frac{\text{Volume of infusion line}}{\text{Total volume in syringe}} \times \text{infusion time (hrs)}$$

The longer the infusion line, the earlier the infusion will end. For example, consider 1 ml and 2 ml infusion lines and a 10 ml syringe volume over a 24 hour period:

$$\frac{1 \text{ ml}}{10 \text{ ml}} \times 24 \text{ hours} = 2 \text{ hours } 24 \text{ mins early}$$

$$\frac{2 \text{ ml}}{10 \text{ ml}} \times 24 \text{ hours} = 4 \text{ hours } 48 \text{ mins early}$$

If the syringe is measured *after* priming, the patient will not receive the prescribed dose:

$$\frac{\text{Volume of infusion line}}{\text{Total volume in syringe}} \times 100\%$$

Again, as the length of the infusion line increases, the actual amount of drug the patient does not receive also increases. For example, consider 1 ml and 2 ml lines and a 10 ml syringe volume over a 24 hour period:

$$\frac{1 \text{ ml}}{10 \text{ ml}} \times 100\% = 10\% \text{ of dose not received}$$

$$\frac{2 \text{ ml}}{10 \text{ ml}} \times 100\% = 20\% \text{ of dose not received}$$

Increasing the volume within the syringe reduces the impact of priming the line, whether performed before or after the length of liquid has been measured:

$$\frac{1 \text{ ml}}{20 \text{ ml}} \times 24 \text{ ml} = 1 \text{ hour } 12 \text{ mins early}$$

$$\frac{1 \text{ ml}}{20 \text{ ml}} \times 100\% = 5\% \text{ of dose not received}$$

Rate setting for MS26:

$$\frac{\text{length of liquid (mm)}}{\text{infusion time (days)}} = \text{rate of infusion (mm/day)}$$

Rate setting for MS16A:

$$\frac{\text{length of liquid (mm)}}{\text{infusion time (hours)}} = \text{rate of infusion (mm/ hour)}$$

Examples are shown below. Note the infusion time for the **MS26** is calculated in **days**; the infusion time for the **MS16A** is calculated in **hours**.

Driver	Length of barrel	Duration of infusion	Rate of infusion
MS26	60 mm	24 hours (1 day)	60 mm/24 hours
	48 mm	12 hours (0.5 days)	96 mm/24 hours
MS16A	48 mm	24 hours	2 mm/hour
	48 mm	12 hours	4 mm/hour

Confusion between the two drivers, in relation to rate setting, has led to fatal errors. The **MS26** is the easier of the two to use; *for infusions of 24 hours, the length of the liquid represents the infusion rate.* The **MS26** offers a greater degree of flexibility, in terms of volume that can be infused, since a longer length of solution, hence volume, can be administered (60 mm over 24 hours). For a 24-hour infusion, the maximum length for the **MS16A** would be 48 mm, due to the practical maximum rate of 2 mm/hour.

5 The syringe is then attached to the driver as shown in Fig. 1.4.

6 Upon insertion of the battery, an alarm will sound. This is the noise the device makes, when:

- the infusion has ended
- the line is blocked
- the start/boost button is depressed for 10 seconds (MS26)
- the start/test button is held down for 5 seconds (MS16A)

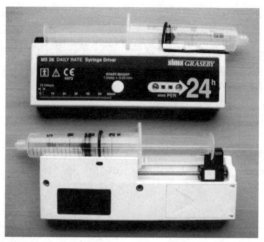

Fig. 1.4 Attaching the syringe to the driver.

7 Press the start button to silence the alarm and to activate the driver. If the light on the front of the driver does not flash (*MS26–every 25 seconds*; *MS16A – every second*), replace the battery. If, during the infusion, the light stops flashing, then the battery is almost depleted. However, the remaining contents of the syringe will be delivered, provided the duration of infusion does not exceed 24 h. The battery can be replaced during the next assembly.

8 Finally, the clear plastic protective cover (as shown in Fig. 1.1) or lockbox (see Fig. 1.2) should be placed over the syringe driver.

9 The syringe and contents should be regularly checked (for example, four hourly within inpatient units); an administration and checking record is suggested (see Appendix 1).

10 An alkaline 9 V battery, as recommended by Graseby, should be able to deliver 50 daily infusions.

It is anticipated that both of these syringe drivers will eventually be withdrawn after the introduction of the Graseby Advancia (see page 15)

(B) Micrel MP daily

The MP daily is very similar to the MS26, in that it delivers the **length of liquid** within the syringe, not the volume, over a 24-h period. It is, however, more sophisticated with definite improvements over the MS drivers:

◆ No boost facility.

◆ More secure and robust syringe attachment.

◆ Infusion rates can be easily fixed, limited, or zoned. If the infusion rate is limited, the upper and the lower limits are applied thereby restricting the rate to a specified range. If the limits are identical, the infusion rate is fixed. If the infusion rate is zoned, the user is alerted to rate settings outside the specifed limits. All serve to reduce the chance of incorrect rate setting.

◆ Once started, the infusion rate cannot be altered (unless the device is turned off and on again).

◆ A range of alarms/warnings to alert the user, for example occlusion alarm, low battery (one infusion remaining), depleted battery, end of plunger travel (i.e. syringe empty; this is set to silence by default), system malfunction, etc.

However, the MP daily retains some of the deficiencies as seen with the MS drivers:

◆ potential confusion (not only with the MS26, but also the MP mlh);

◆ no alarm upon removal of the syringe, or when siphoning occurs.

The MP daily can deliver a maximum length of 60 mm per infusion (this represents the maximum distance that the syringe plunger can be extended and still fit on the device); the rate varies from 1–99 mm per 24 h. By having a rate of delivery based upon length of fluid, greater flexibility in the choice of syringe (brand and size) is permitted. Again, only Luer Lok^{TM} syringes should be used. Syringes of varying sizes can be attached to the MP Daily, with 30 ml possibly being the largest, without the device being adjusted by the manufacturer.

With a 30 ml sized syringe, a liquid length of 60 mm equates to approximately 25 ml. Hence, the largest volume of liquid that can be infused is approximately 25 ml. The manufacturer can adjust the syringe fixing strap to allow up to 60 ml syringes to be attached (but only 60 mm liquid length can be infused).

The MP daily defaults to a line priming function. This can only be used when the syringe is attached, just after the device has been activated and before the rate is set. It may be sensible to disable the priming function for the following reasons:

◆ It may cause confusion with rate setting. The general consensus is to prime the line, then calculate the delivery rate, thereby, ensuring that the infusion lasts for the desired duration (see Box 1.1). It seems pointless to attach the syringe to prime the line and then detach it, in order to measure the length of fluid remaining.

◆ There is a possibility that the priming function may be activated accidentally during the setup procedure.

Assembly

1 Turn the device on, by depressing both chevron buttons, until the device beeps. The previous infusion rate now flashes on the display.

2 Fill the syringe with the prescribed drug(s) and dilute the contents up to a maximum length of 60 mm. Use the millimetre scale on the driver for reference.

3 Prime the infusion line, if required, *before* measuring and attaching the syringe. (Note—may be advisable to disable the device's priming function.)

4 Measure the length of barrel against the millimetre scale on the syringe driver as shown in Fig. 1.5.

5 Attach the syringe to the device as shown in Fig. 1.6.

6 Set the delivery rate. This is derived by dividing the length of the liquid by the required infusion time.

$$\frac{\text{length of liquid (mm)}}{\text{infusion time (days)}} = \text{rate of infusion (mm/day)}$$

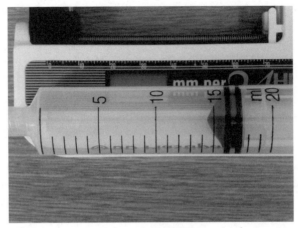

Fig. 1.5 Measuring the syringe on the MP daily.

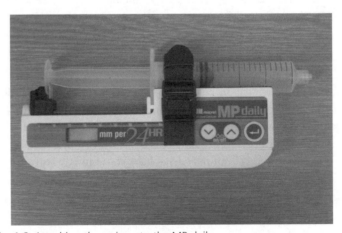

Fig. 1.6 Attaching the syringe to the MP daily.

Examples are shown below. Note the infusion time for the MP daily is calculated in **days**.

Length of barrel	Duration of Infusion	Rate of Infusion
60 mm	24 h (1 day)	60 mm/24 h
48 mm	12 h (0.5 days)	96 mm/24 h

The rate of infusion is set by using the two chevron buttons (increase or decrease). The infusion starts after the 'enter' button is pressed for three seconds. Two horizontal bars on the LCD flash, to confirm that the infusion is running. Note that once the infusion has started, the rate cannot be changed. If the low battery alarm sounds during the infusion (and a battery sign is shown in the LCD), any button can be depressed to silence it. The batteries will need replacing before commencing the next infusion.

7 The syringe and contents should be checked regularly (for example, four hourly within in-patient units); an administration and checking record is suggested (see Appendix 1).

8 The device uses six AAA 1.5 V alkaline batteries. These will last for approximately 50 infusions (up to two months, if used for daily infusions).

(C) Micrel MP mlh

The MP mlh is a portable battery operated syringe driver that differs from all the similar current devices on the market (in the UK) in that it delivers at a rate determined by millilitres per hour (ml/h). It is currently only calibrated to deliver a continuous infusion with a 20 ml BD Plastipak syringe, although the software may be improved to increase the variety of size and brand. Its appearance, dimensions, battery life, and alarm functions are similar to the MP daily (see Fig. 1.1); it is also more sophisticated than the MS drivers with definite improvements:

◆ No boost facility.

◆ More secure and robust syringe attachment.

- A range of alarms/warnings to alert the user, for example occlusion alarm, low battery (one infusion remaining), depleted battery, end of plunger travel (i.e. syringe empty), system malfunction.

The setup procedure is similar to the MP daily, except that the rate is set in ml/h. Unlike the Advancia MS, the rate has to be calculated manually:

$$\frac{\text{volume in syringe (ml)}}{\text{infusion time (h)}} = \text{rate of infusion (ml/h)}$$

This device, in its current configuration, is probably unsuitable for use in the palliative care setting.

- The infusion rate can be altered during the course of the infusion. This is unlikely to be of any benefit in the palliative care setting; in fact, it is more likely to be a hazard.

- There are no configurable options (such as alarms, infusion rate limits) unlike the MP daily.

- Currently, the device is limited to a volume of 20 ml and a specific brand of syringe.

(D) Graseby Advancia MS

Important note This device is presently experimental and may not enter production.

The four devices discussed above are very similar in weight and dimensions which make them very suitable for ambulatory use. However, there remains the potential for confusion between all four devices and they all lack suitable alarms (notably syringe displacement and siphoning). The Advancia has been designed to meet all current legislation and safety requirements. These benefits, though, may have been offset by the increase in size and weight of the device (see Fig. 1.1). Certainly a weight of 600 g may well reduce its suitability for some palliative care patients.

Upon first appearance, this device appears complicated, particularly when compared to the MS26 and MS16. In order to comply with the current legislation and safety demands, technological advances have been incorporated into the Advancia's design. The device has several advantages over the other four:

◆ Comprehensive alarm system, including syringe displacement
◆ Infusion rate set automatically
◆ Tampering becomes much harder
◆ Syringe unlikely to become dislodged by accidental action
◆ Many configurable infusion options, making this a flexible device

However, these advances have been at the expense of other features and there are potential problems:

◆ The Advancia is more than 3 times as heavy as the other devices
◆ Battery life is greatly reduced (see Fig. 1.1) making this a more expensive device to run
◆ The device is not foolproof and there is the potential for user error (particularly in the selection of brand of syringe—see setup below).
◆ There needs to be a significant education and training programme before this device can be entered into service, especially in the palliative care setting.

Assembly

1 Switch syringe driver on and wait for self-test to be completed. The device displays 'NEW PATIENT?' when ready.

2 Draw up medication and prime the infusion line.

3 Lift the barrel clamp and insert the syringe into the attachment, firmly pushing it into both provided slots. The attachment will spring shut and a beep confirms that the syringe is correctly in place. To secure the syringe, close the barrel clamp.

4 Insert infusion line's safety clip into the allotted slot.

5 The screen will display the syringe brand last confirmed, and the size of the syringe that the pump has detected. Confirm the brand, and size, or change using the appropriate buttons.

6 Close the cover to secure the infusion line's safety clip and syringe.

7 Program the syringe driver. The device currently displays 'NEW PATIENT?' For a new patient, press the 'YES' button. Enter the volume to be infused, followed by the infusion time (in hours, then minutes).

8 Lock the cover and press the green start button to initiate the infusion.

Risk management is clearly an issue with these devices, particularly as errors (occasionally fatal) are still reported. It is recommended that only one type of driver is available per site, preferably the MS26 or the MP daily, due to their relative simplicity but clearly this is not always possible. In situations where different syringe drivers are available, it would be prudent to fix the rates of infusion. For example, the length of liquid in the syringe should be fixed to 48 mm. The rates of infusion of the devices remain fixed at 48 mm/24 h (MS26 and MP daily) and 2 mm/h (MS16A). There should also be a clear programme of staff training and education. Additionally, and where ever possible, the syringe and its contents should be checked regularly (e.g. four hourly, within in-patient units); an administration and checking record is suggested (see Appendix 1).

Infusion site

The site of infusion has implications for the patient. If the patient is ambulatory, then the chest or abdomen are the preferred sites. Previously, the upper aspect of the arm was considered to be the first choice. However, movement of the arm may lead to the development of problems, such as bruising. If the patient is distressed, the placement of the site around the scapula will reduce the likelihood of the patient accidentally removing it. Occasionally, the thigh may be used. Rotation of the site, every three days, should be routine in order to minimize site reactions. In some patients, this may not be feasible and health professionals should monitor the infusion site carefully and re-site as required.

Infusion site reactions

Local site reactions are occasionally encountered problems with CSCIs. There have been many suggested causes of site reactions:[6]

- Glass particles from the ampoule
- Infection
- Sterile abscess
- Allergic response to nickel needle
- Chemical reaction in subcutaneous tissue
- Tonicity of solution
- pH

A recent unpublished study[7] suggested that site reactions are more likely to occur, if the site is older than 72 hours, or the infusion contains cyclizine, high doses of diamorphine, or levomepromazine. Indeed increasing doses of diamorphine have previously been linked to site reactions.[6] The following step-wise approach should be considered in order to prevent the development of site reactions:

- *Dilute the solution as much as practical* (a 20 ml syringe is the recommended minimum size; a 12-hourly infusion may be required), but ensure the solution is as close to physiological tonicity as possible. Both hypotonic and hypertonic solutions can give rise to site reactions. Water for Injections (WFI) is hypotonic; sodium chloride 0.9% (NaCl) is isotonic. The osmolality of 21 different solutions containing one or more drugs commonly used in palliative care has been investigated.[8] The study found that all solutions had an osmolality, the same or less, than NaCl. Therefore, if dilution is necessary, **NaCl** should be used. There are two exceptions when WFI must be used:

  - solutions containing cyclizine (crystals of cyclizine hydrochloride form in the presence of chloride ions[9]) and,
  - solutions of high concentrations of diamorphine (diamorphine precipitates in NaCl at concentrations >40 mg/ml[10,11]).

- *Rotate the site at least every 72 hours.* In certain situations (e.g. methadone infusions) the site may need to be rotated daily.

- *Use a non-metal cannula.* Several studies have examined the use of non-metal cannulae versus metal butterfly needles.[12–14] The duration of the subcutaneous infusion site was extended significantly with non-metal cannulae in all studies. This conclusion was confirmed in a recent review.[15]

- *Consider changing the drug combination,* for example if high dose diamorphine is believed to be the cause of the reaction, alfentanil may be considered.
- *Hyaluronidase*—there is little evidence for using hyaluronidase in order to prevent the development of site reactions. Its use has been suggested in lieu of its use for hypodermoclysis, although the use of hyaluronidase may contribute to poor tolerance of a CSCI. Doses used for this indication range from 150 units per 500 ml infusion fluid to 250 units per 500 ml infusion fluid.[16–18] Given the maximum volume likely to be infused via a CSCI is smaller than for hypodermoclysis, the maximum dose of hyaluronidase that is recommended is 150 units per site.
- *Dexamethasone 1 mg.* Use of dexamethasone in syringe drivers to attenuate site reactions is a complex issue. There are unreported anecdotes describing success and a case report has suggested benefits in improving the tolerance of subcutaneous methadone infusions.[19] Recently, a study concluded that the use of low-dose dexamethasone for such an indication increased the longevity of subcutaneous sites.[20] Nonetheless, dexamethasone is clearly associated with many concentration-dependent incompatibility issues with drugs such as cyclizine, haloperidol, levomepromazine, and promethazine, as shown in Chapter 4. Understanding the nature of these incompatibilities can help to determine whether addition of dexamethasone is of benefit, or of detriment. There are at least two possible explanations for the apparent efficacy of low-dose dexamethasone in attenuation of site reactions: its anti-inflammatory effect, or the possibility that the concentration of the offending drug is effectively reduced by a chemical reaction.

With this in mind, it is useful to discuss some potential outcomes when drugs are mixed in syringe driver solutions. The best confirmation of stability and compatibility will always be the performance of an appropriate laboratory analysis to examine the range of concentrations commonly used, prepared in the usual diluents and stored over a range of temperatures, reflecting use in the clinical situation. The presence of a precipitate on mixing of drugs is a simple way of identifying an incompatibility. Sometimes, however, solutions can either remain clear when drugs are mixed (even though a chemical reaction may have taken place), or a precipitate may initially form as a result of a chemical reaction, but dissolve upon agitation. Hence, a clear, colourless solution, free from precipitate is not a definitive proof of compatibility or stability of any of the drugs in the admixture. In a recent study,[21] it was shown that even when an admixture of dexamethasone and midazolam prepared in normal saline remained clear, there was a significant loss of midazolam over 48 h with only 60–80% of the initial concentration of midazolam remaining in syringes stored at 35–39°C.

Most drugs are formulated as salts of weak acids or weak bases, in order to improve solubility (an example of a drug in its salt form is morphine sulphate—this is the salt of the relatively insoluble weak base, morphine). Different salts of these weak acids or bases may exhibit different solubilities, with some salts of the same drug being more soluble than others (e.g. morphine tartrate is more soluble than morphine sulphate; cyclizine lactate is more soluble than cyclizine hydrochloride). Manufacturers will select the most suitable salt for the purpose of their formulations and often the salt chosen is that with the highest solubility.

The solubility of a given drug can also be influenced by the pH of the solution. If the pH is changed, for example, by addition of another drug solution, precipitation of the actual weak acid or base can occur. Diamorphine hydrochloride shows pH-dependent solubility in NaCl; the pH must remain below 6.0 for the diamorphine salt to remain in solution.[10,11]

When dexamethasone is added to several drug solutions, there is often an initial cloudiness, or turbidity (precipitation). Upon agitation, the turbidity may disappear and the solution is infused; if the turbidity remains, the mixture is clearly physically incompatible. There are two possible explanations for this effect; one that supports the use of dexamethasone for attenuation of site reactions (pH effect), whilst the other opposes its use (chemical reaction).

The first explanation involves pH and solubility. Issues with pH are likely to occur when two injections (or more) of widely differing pH are mixed. pH ranges for many different injections used in palliative care are clearly illustrated in the monographs in Chapter 2. The pH of dexamethasone injection may range from 7 to 8.5 while the pH values for many commonly used injections are in the pH range from 2 to 6. This effect of pH on solubility is usually seen as turbidity. Occasionally, there may be transient "local cloudiness" when dexamethasone is initially added, but this disappears on mixing. This effect may be due to a momentary large change in pH in the area where the dexamethasone solution is being placed; once the solution mixes, however, the pH change overall is minimized and the drugs remain in solution (the solution remains clear). Assuming this to be the case, the solution is therefore safe to infuse and the patient will receive the prescribed medication. It does, however, highlight that there may be potential problems at higher concentrations (such as we see with dexamethasone and midazolam; at certain lower concentrations, a clear solution results but at higher concentrations, a precipitate will remain).

A chemical reaction between drugs and/or excipients is another potential outcome, when two or more drug solutions are mixed. Such a reaction may occur upon addition of dexamethasone to a drug solution. The resulting solution may be clear and free from precipitation if the compound produced is soluble. For example, this occurs when dexamethasone and glycopyrronium are mixed together; a hydrolysis reaction produces a water soluble product. If a poorly soluble product is formed by the reaction, it may initially precipitate and produce the transient 'local cloudiness' mentioned above; but upon agitation, the precipitate may dissolve. This can give a false impression that the combination is stable. Should the compound produced by this reaction have little pharmacological activity, a lack of clinical effect may be noticed. There is, of course, the potential for the formation of a soluble, possible toxic compound.

The definitive technique to determine whether a combination is stable or not is by laboratory analysis. Clinical practicality may necessitate the use of low-dose dexamethasone in combination with other drugs, in situations of continued site intolerance, despite the measures already mentioned. If a combination produces crystallization or precipitation, then this clearly should not be given and alternative methods must be found. If the solution remains clear, or if there is only transient turbidity, then, in the absence of laboratory data, clinical outcome can be used, provisionally, to determine whether the mixture is chemically stable, until such time that analytical data on stability and compatibility are available. A practical solution to circumvent the incompatibility issues involves the injection of dexamethasone directly into the infusion site, with a small volume (e.g. 0.5 ml) of NaCl being used as a flush prior to the commencement of the CSCI.

Frequently asked questions

1 What diluent should be used to dilute drug mixtures?

Any of the following three diluents are suitable for subcutaneous infusions: NaCl, WFI, dextrose 5% in water (DEX). In most cases, the diluent used should be NaCl, which is chosen to ensure the solution is as close to physiological tonicity as possible. The main exceptions to this rule are solutions containing cyclizine, or diamorphine at a concentration greater than 40 mg/ml, in which case, WFI should be used. Drug infusions not containing cyclizine that cause site irritation (e.g. mixtures containing methadone or levomepromazine) should be diluted with NaCl. The Drug Information and Compatibility Chapters describe, where applicable, the diluents that can be used.

2 When should the syringe driver be started?

When converting a patient from a modified release (m/r) preparation of an oral opioid (e.g. morphine, hydromorphone, or oxycodone) to a CSCI, there is no need for a crossover period; it may be started at the time of the next dosage. For practical purposes, this is often the best method. However; in order to achieve or maintain adequate analgesia, it may be necessary to administer a suitable 'rescue' dose of subcutaneous opioid. Note that some centres usually start the CSCI some four hours before the next oral dose is due.

If a CSCI is required for a patient on transdermal fentanyl or buprenorphine, it is currently considered the best practice to leave this *in situ*. Refer to Chapter 3, Symptom Control with the Syringe Driver, for further details.

3 When should the CSCI be stopped, if oral treatment is to continue?

The CSCI should be stopped as soon as the oral m/r dose of opioid is given. No crossover period is necessary since the m/r preparations provide an 'immediate' release dose. However, ensure that appropriate breakthrough medication has been prescribed.

4 When should the CSCI be stopped if a transdermal fentanyl or buprenorphine patch is applied?

The CSCI should be stopped 12 hours after the patch has been applied.

5 What is the usual number of drugs that can be mixed together?

Before mixing drugs together, it is important to check for stability information. This book has an extensive list of mixtures in Chapter 4; other sources of information include, the local Medicines Information Centre (NHS hospitals, UK), or the Internet (e.g. www.palliativedrugs.com, www.pallcare.info).

It is common to see at least two or three drugs mixed in the same syringe; occasionally four may be required. In fact, most of the symptoms encountered at the end of life, can be controlled effectively by the use of only four drugs:

Analgesic (e.g. diamorphine, morphine)

Sedative (e.g. clonazepam, midazolam)

Anticholinergic (e.g. glycopyrronium, hyoscine hydrobromide)

Antiemetic (e.g. cyclizine, dimenhydrinate)

These drugs have been shown to be physically compatible at usual concentrations. (Refer to cyclizine and diamorphine monographs in Chapter 2 for known incompatibility issues.)

6 What can be done to minimize stability problems?

The mixture should be diluted to the maximum volume and be delivered over a maximum time of 24 hours because chemical stability cannot be assured after this time. To further reduce the risk of incompatibility, the contents of the syringe driver and giving set should be protected from direct sunlight (especially mixtures containing levomepromazine). Temperature can also affect the stability of mixtures. Simple measures, such as ensuring that the driver is placed on top of bed covers, rather than in them, could reduce the effects of temperature.

Certain incompatible mixtures are known to be dependent upon concentration (e.g. cyclizine and diamorphine). The risk of crystallization or precipitation may be overcome by using more dilute

12 hourly infusions. However, to ensure that the rate setting is correct, consult a palliative care specialist in this situation.

7 What can be done if a syringe driver is unavailable?

This is a fairly common problem encountered in hospitals in the UK. As a short-term measure, CSCIs can be administered by utilizing other syringe pumps, with the solution in the syringe being diluted to a suitable volume (e.g. 48 ml). These devices usually deliver at a rate of **ml/hour**. Alternatively, a butterfly needle may be sited subcutaneously and bolus injections can be given, as necessary, to cover the period until a driver becomes available. It would be wise to check with a Palliative Care Specialist before proceeding.

References

1. Wright BM, Callan K. Slow drug infusions using a portable syringe driver. *Br Med J* 1979; **2**(6190):582.

2. Russel PS. Analgesia in terminal malignant disease. *Br Med J* 1979; **1**(6177):1561.

3. David J. A survey of the use of syringe drivers in Marie Curie Centres. *Eur J Cancer Care* 1992; **1**:23–28.

4. Herndon CM, Fike DS. Continuous subcutaneous infusion practices of United States Hospices. *J Pain Symptom Manage* 2001; **22**:1027–1034.

5. Medicines and Healthcare products Regulatory Agency. Evaluation 02152 http://nww.mda.nhs.uk/pumpevaluation 2003.

6. Oliver D. The Tonicity of Solutions used in Continuous Subcutaneous Infusions. The Cause of Skin Reactions? *Hospital Pharmacy Practice* 1991; Sept:158–164.

7. Pickard J. Manchester, UK. Personal Communication 2004.

8. Schneider JJ, Wilson KM, Ravenscroft PJ. A study of the osmolality and pH of subcutaneous drug infusion solutions. *Aust J Hosp Pharm* 1997; **27**(1):29–31.

9. Grassby PF, Hutchings L. Drug combinations in syringe drivers: the compatibility and stability of diamorphine with cyclizine and haloperidol. *Palliat Med* 1997; **11**:217–224.

10. Page J, Hudson SA. Diamorphine hydrochloride compatibility with saline. *Pharm J* 1982; **228**:238–239.

11. Hain WR, Kirk B. Stability of diamorphine-sodium chloride solutions. *Anaesthesia* 1985; **40**:1241.

12. Macmillan K, Bruera E, Kuehn N, Selmser P, Macmillan A. A prospective comparison study between a butterfly needle and a Teflon cannula for subcutaneous narcotic administration. *J Pain Symptom Manage* 1994; **9**(2):82–84.

13. Ross JR, Saunders Y, Cochrane M, Zeppetella G. A prospective, within-patient comparison between metal butterfly needles and Teflon cannulae in subcutaneous infusion of drugs to terminally ill hospice patients. *Palliat Med* 2002; **16**(1):13–16.

14. Dawkins L, Britton D, Johnson I, Higgins B, Dean T. A randomised trial of winged Vialon cannulae and metal butterfly needles. *Int J Palliat Nurs* 2000; **6**(3):110–116.

15. Torre MC. Subcutaneous infusion: non-metal cannulae vs metal butterfly needles. *Br J Community Nurs* 2002; **7**(7):365–369.

16. Bruera E, Legris MA, Kuehn N, Miller MJ. Hypodermoclysis for the administration of fluids and narcotic analgesics in patients with advanced cancer. *J Pain Symptom Manage* 1990; **5**(4):218–220.

17. Constans T, Dutertre JP, Froge E. Hypodermoclysis in dehydrated elderly patients: local effects with and without hyaluronidase. *J Palliat Care* 1991; **7**(2):10–12.

18. Bruera E, Neumann CM, Pituskin E, Calder K, Hanson J. A randomised controlled trial of local injections of hyaluronidase versus placebo in cancer patients receiving subcutaneous hydration. *Ann Oncol* 1999; **10**(10):1255–1258.

19. Mathew P, Storey P. Subcutaneous methadone in terminally ill patients: manageable local toxicity. *J Pain Symptom Manage* 1999; **18**:49–52.

20. Reymond L, Charles MA, Bowman J, Treston P. The effect of dexamethasone on the longevity of syringe driver subcutaneous sites in palliative care patients. *MJA* 2003; **178**:486–489.

21. Good P, Schneider J, Ravenscroft P. The compatibility and stability of midazolam and dexamethasone in infusion solutions. *J Pain Symptom Manage* 2004; **27**:471–475.

Chapter 2

Drug information

Introduction

During the last few years, it has become evident that a greater number of drugs are being administered by a CSCI. Although the drugs included here have product licences, the majority of these drugs (see Table 2.1) are unlicensed for administration via a CSCI. However, most pharmaceutical companies will be aware that such 'off label' use occurs.

Most drug combinations used in palliative care form clear, colourless solutions, that are free from precipitation or crystallization. However, this does not confirm stability because invisible chemical reactions may occur. For example, dexamethasone and glycopyrronium mix to form a clear, colourless solution that is free from precipitation. However, an unseen chemical reaction occurs and the effectiveness of the combination may be reduced.

Table 2.1 Drugs that can be given by continuous subcutaneous infusion

Alfentanil	Fentanyl	Levomepromazine	Phenobarbital
Clonazepam	Glycopyrronium	Methadone	Promethazine
Cyclizine	Haloperidol	Metoclopramide	Ranitidine
Dexamethasone	Hydromorphone	Midazolam	Sufentanil
Diamorphine	Hyoscine butylbromide	Morphine	Tramadol
Diclofenac	Hyoscine hydrobromide	Octreotide	
Dihydrocodeine	Ketamine	Ondansetron	
Dimenhydrinate	Ketorolac	Oxycodone	

One of the most useful predictors of drug compatibility is pH. This can affect the solubility of drugs and chemical stability of the mixture. The majority of drugs given by CSCI are acidic, with only dexamethasone, diclofenac, ketorolac, and phenobarbital, being alkaline. Consequently, combinations involving these drugs tend to be incompatible and separate infusions are usually recommended. The pH values of individual drugs are included in the following monographs. There are, however, several other factors that can affect the stability of drug mixtures, for example concentration, temperature, and exposure to sunlight.

The following monographs refer to drugs that are available in the UK *unless,* otherwise stated. Where possible, references to drug availability in Australia (AUS) and the USA have been made.

Opioid analgesics

There are several opioid analgesics that can be administered via a CSCI. One of the commonly encountered problems involves the conversion of one opioid to another, for example, oral oxycodone to subcutaneous diamorphine or morphine. Table 2.2, overleaf, provides conversion factors from several different opioids and routes to subcutaneous diamorphine.[1–10,62,64] Table 2.3 provides a more comprehensive dose equivalence chart and Table 2.4 shows the conversion factors for several different opioids for conversion to subcutaneous morphine.

Important note Equianalgesic doses are difficult to ascertain due to wide inter-patient variations. Initial dose conversions should be conservative; it is preferable to under-dose the patient and use rescue medication for any shortfalls.

Table 2.2 Opioid conversion factors—**diamorphine**

Opioid dose (in milligrams)	Conversion factor to subcutaneous diamorphine* (in milligrams)
Alfentanil (parenteral)	10
Buprenorphine (buccal)	†
Buprenorphine (transdermal)	Refer to Table 2.3
Codeine (oral)	0.04
Diamorphine (oral)	0.33
Dihydrocodeine (oral)	0.04
Dihydrocodeine (subcutaneous)	0.15
Dipipanone (oral)	0.17
Fentanyl (parenteral)	30–50
Fentanyl (transdermal)	Refer to Table 2.3
Hydromorphone (oral)	2.5
Hydromorphone (parenteral)	5–6.6
Methadone (oral)	‡
Morphine (oral)	0.33
Morphine (parenteral)	0.66–1.0
Oxycodone (oral)	0.5
Oxycodone (parenteral)	0.66
Tramadol (oral and parenteral)	0.08¶

*Multiply the opioid dose by the conversion factor to give the equivalent subcutaneous diamorphine dose.
e.g. Oral morphine 120 mg.

†Buprenorphine is a partial agonist. Converting to another opioid after long term buccal use will be difficult. A palliative care or pain specialist must be consulted.

‡Methadone has a prolonged half-life that can result in accumulation with repeated doses. A palliative care or pain specialist should be consulted.

¶Caution should be applied when transferring a patient on tramadol to a strong opioid. The analgesia produced by tramadol is only weakly related to its opioid agonist property. Nonetheless, upon multiple dosing, oral tramadol appears to be bioequivalent to parenteral since oral studies show a 4:1 tramadol:morphine potency, whilst IV studies show an 8-10:1 tramadol:morphine potency (i.e. ratio doubles due to the increase in bioavailability of parenteral morphine over oral).

Table 2.3 Dose equivalence chart

12-hourly oral Morphine (mg)	24-hourly oral Morphine (mg)	12-hourly oral Oxycodone (mg)	Transdermal Fentanyl (micrograms/h)	Transdermal Buprenorphine (mg)	Diamorphine* SC 4 hourly (mg)	Diamorphine* CSCI in 24 hr (mg)	Alfentanil SC PRN (mg)	Alfentanil CSCI in 24 hr (mg)
10		5		35	2.5	5–10	0.25	0.5–1
15	30	5–10		35	2.5	10	0.25	1
30	60	15	25	52.5	5	20	0.5	2
60	120	30	25–50	70	5–10	40	0.5–1	4
90	180	40	50	105	10	60	1	6
120	240	60	50–75	140	15	80	1.5	8
150	300	70	75–100		15–20	100	1.5–2	10
180	360	90	100		20	120	2	12
200	400	100	125		20	130	2	13
240	490	120	125–150		20–30	160	2–3	16
260	540	130	150		30	190	3	19
300	600	150	150–175		30	200	3	20
330	660	160	175		30–40	220	3–4	22
360	720	180	200		40	240	4	24
420	840	200	225–250		40–50	290	4–5	29
480	960	240	250–275		50–60	330	5–6	33
540	1080	250	300		60	360	6	36

*Parenteral diamorphine is considered to be 1.5 times more potent than morphine and oxycodone (i.e. diamorphine 10 mg = oxycodone 15 mg = morphine 15 mg)

Table 2.4 Opioid conversion factors—**morphine**

Opioid dose (in milligrams)	Conversion factor to subcutaneous morphine* (in milligrams)
Codeine (oral)	0.03
Fentanyl (parenteral)	100
Fentanyl (transdermal)	Refer to manufacturer's table to calculate equivalent morphine oral dose then convert to daily subcutaneous dose by dividing by 3
Hydromorphone (oral)	2.5–3.5
Hydromorphone (parenteral)	5–7.5
Methadone (oral)	†
Morphine (oral)	0.33–0.5
Oxycodone (oral)	0.5–1.0
Tramadol (oral and parenteral)	0.125‡
Sufentanil	¶

*Multiply the opioid dose by the conversion factor to give the equivalent subcutaneous morphine dose.
e.g. oxycodone 30 mg bd = 60 mg x 0.5 = 30 mg subcutaneous **morphine daily**

†Methadone has a prolonged half-life that can result in accumulation with repeated doses. A palliative care or pain specialist should be consulted.

‡Caution should be applied when transferring a patient on tramadol to a strong opioid. The analgesia produced by tramadol is only weakly related to its opioid agonist property. Nonetheless, upon multiple dosing, oral tramadol appears to be bioequivalent to parenteral since oral studies show a 4:1 tramadol:morphine potency, whilst IV studies show an 8-10:1 tramadol:morphine potency (i.e. ratio doubles due to the increase in bioavailability of parenteral morphine over oral).

¶There are no comparative data; a specialist should be approached for this information. However, sufentanil is stated to be 7 to 10 times more potent than fentanyl.

Alfentanil

Specialist palliative care input recommended.

Usual dose: Providing titration occurs correctly, the dose of alfentanil can be increased as necessary. The initial dose depends upon the patient's previous opioid treatment (see Table 2.3 for diamorphine equivalents). For opioid naïve patients, a suitable starting dose would be 0.5–1mg over 24 hours. If pain is uncontrolled, the dose can be increased by 30–50%. Rescue doses must be available for breakthrough pain, although the optimum dosing schedule is currently unknown because alfentanil has a short duration of action. However, it is suggested that one sixth of the daily dose is given every 1-2 hours. If more than three rescue doses are required for breakthrough pain (*not* incident pain—see page 100) in a 24-hour period, the total daily dose in the CSCI should be increased by 30%.

Preparations: UK: 1 mg/2 ml; 5 mg/10 ml; 5 mg/ml. Schedule 2 controlled drug.

AUS: 1 mg/2 ml; 5 mg/10 ml. Schedule 8 controlled drug.

USA: 1 mg/2 ml; 2.5 mg/5 ml; 5 mg/10 ml; 10 mg/20 ml. Schedule 2 controlled drug.

Diluent: Dilute with NaCl. WFI or DEX may also be used.

pH: 4.0–6.0.

Information: Alfentanil is a synthetic opioid, with strong agonist activity at μ- and κ-receptors. It is chemically related to fentanyl and is more lipophilic than morphine. Alfentanil is a suitable alternative to diamorphine for use in a CSCI, particularly in patients with renal failure. It is routinely used in surgical procedures as an analgesic and adjunct to general anaesthetics. Alfentanil is approximately 10 times as potent as diamorphine (given subcutaneously)[3] and one quarter as potent as fentanyl.[11]

Alfentanil is extensively metabolized in the liver by the CYP3A4 isoenzyme to inactive compounds, with a mean elimination half-life of 90 minutes. Drugs that reduce hepatic blood flow or interfere with this enzyme could alter responses to alfentanil, e.g. drugs such as protease inhibitors, diltiazem, ketoconazole, cimetidine, clarithromycin, and erythromycin may increase the effect of alfentanil; drugs such as carbamazepine, phenobarbital, and phenytoin may reduce the effect of alfentanil. Note that although patients requiring a CSCI of alfentanil are unlikely to be using most of these drugs, their effect on alfentanil metabolism may persist for several days even after cessation. The effects of co-existing liver disease may necessitate an empirical dosage reduction in order to avoid symptoms of opioid toxicity. A dosage reduction in obese patients may also be required. Dosage adjustments are usually **not** required in renal failure.[12,13]

One study[14] suggested that tolerance to the analgesic efficacy of alfentanil could develop relatively rapidly, which would limit its use in chronic treatment. However, another more recent study provided no evidence of tolerance to opioids.[15] Further work needs to be performed to determine the significance and incidence of this potential problem for all the opioids.

Alfentanil appears to be physically stable with most drugs used in the syringe driver (see Chapter 4) except cyclizine. As with diamorphine, the hydrochloride salt of alfentanil can cause crystallization with cyclizine as concentrations increase. Any mixtures with cyclizine should be diluted with WFI and closely checked for signs of crystallisation. Alfentanil has been shown to be physically and chemically compatible with midazolam[16] and ondansetron under stated conditions in NaCl.[17]

Clonazepam

Usual dose: 1 mg to 4 mg over 24 hours. Doses up to 8 mg can be used to treat terminal agitation. Clonazepam has a long half-life and may be given as a stat subcutaneous injection, rather than CSCI (volume permitting).

Diluent: Although the product is supplied with 1 ml of WFI, NaCl or DEX can be used to dilute a CSCI.

Preparations: 1 mg/ml in solvent with 1ml WFI to be added. Not available in the USA.

pH: 3.4–4.3.

Information: Clonazepam is a benzodiazepine derivative with anti-epileptic properties. It is extensively metabolized in the liver to possibly weakly acting metabolites and the cytochrome CYP3A pathway appears to be important.[18] Drugs that interfere with this enzyme could alter responses to clonazepam, e.g. drugs such as protease inhibitors, diltiazem, ketoconazole, cimetidine, clarithromycin, and erythromycin may increase the effect of clonazepam; drugs such as carbamazepine, phenobarbital, and phenytoin may reduce the effect of clonazepam. Note that, although patients requiring a CSCI of clonazepam are unlikely to be using most of these drugs, their effect on its metabolism may persist for several days after cessation. This is likely to be of significance when transferring a patient from an oral anti-epileptic.

Clonazepam has several uses in palliative care:

- Neuropathic pain
- Terminal agitation
- Anxiety
- Myoclonus
- Seizures
- Intractable hiccup

Occasionally, a patient with neuropathic pain may require a syringe driver towards the end of his/her life. Aside from ketamine and methadone, most recognized adjuvant analgesia cannot be given via CSCI. If left untreated, the neuropathic pain may manifest as terminal restlessness. Clonazepam can be used both orally and subcutaneously for the treatment of neuropathic pain. However, there are no randomized trials supporting the use of clonazepam in cancer-related neuropathic pain, or for administration via CSCI, although a recent case series reported its use.[19] Nonetheless, it is an accepted treatment in several centres and there are anecdotal reports in the literature relating to non-malignant neuropathic pain and use via CSCI.[20–23]

Clonazepam is an alternative to midazolam, but should be reserved for the treatment of terminal restlessness, associated with a previous history of neuropathic pain, or where the volume of injection associated with midazolam is too great (e.g. clonazepam may be the preferred sedative for patients receiving oxycodone via CSCI).

It has been shown that adsorption onto PVC infusion sets occurs with clonazepam injection. [24,25] The clinical significance of this effect is yet to be determined, although one study [24] suggested that this should be of little significance. However, a recent study has shown that significant loss of clonazepam does occur when infused through PVC tubing over 24 hours. Use of non-PVC tubing solved this problem.[26]

Reports suggest that clonazepam is physically compatible with haloperidol, hyoscine hydrobromide and morphine sulphate.[23,27] Refer to Chapter 4 for further compatibility data.

Cyclizine

Usual dose: 100 to 150 mg over 24 hours.

Diluent: WFI, or DEX. NaCl must **not** be used

Preparations: 50 mg/ml. Available in Australia only through the SAS Scheme (see Appendix 2). Unavailable in the USA.

pH: 3.3–3.7.

Information: Cyclizine is an antihistamine with additional antimuscarinic activity. It is metabolized in the liver to a relatively inactive metabolite.[18] It should be used with caution in patients with glaucoma, although this is not a contra-indication for patients with advanced disease.

Cyclizine is a useful antiemetic, if the cause of nausea or vomiting is due to stimulation of the vomiting centre (e.g. by radiotherapy to the head and neck, raised intracranial pressure) or vagus nerve (e.g. bowel obstruction with colic). Is also useful if nausea and vomiting is worse on movement. This drug is implicated in many compatibility problems. Cyclizine may precipitate as the concentration of chloride ions increase or if the pH is greater than 6.8.[28,29] There is a theoretical risk of precipitation with drugs that are formulated in a solution containing chloride ions. Such drugs include alfentanil, diamorphine, metoclopramide and oxycodone. In addition, there are known concentration-dependent compatibility issues with alfentanil, dexamethasone, diamorphine, hyoscine butylbromide, metoclopramide and oxycodone.

Cyclizine lactate and diamorphine hydrochloride mixtures are chemically and physically stable in WFI up to concentrations of 20 mg/ml over 24 hours. If the diamorphine concentration exceeds 20 mg/ml, crystallization may occur unless the concentration of cyclizine is *no greater than* 10 mg/ml. Similarly, if the concentration of cyclizine exceeds 20 mg/ml, crystallization may occur unless the concentration of diamorphine is *no greater than* 15 mg/ml.[28] See Chapter 4 for further drug compatibility data.

Undesirable effects include drowsiness, dry mouth, urinary retention, and restlessness. These are more common with higher doses.

Rarely, aggravation of severe heart failure may occur and extrapyramidal reactions have also been reported. Cyclizine may occasionally cause irritation at the injection site.

Dexamethasone

Important note A recent change in product labelling in the UK has caused some confusion. Dexamethasone is formulated as dexamethasone sodium phosphate; it is available as a 10 mg/2 ml vial, i.e. 10 mg dexamethasone sodium phosphate in 2 ml. This is roughly equivalent to 8 mg/2 ml of dexamethasone. In order to avoid administration issues, doctors are encouraged to prescribe parenteral dexamethasone in terms of the sodium phosphate salt, so:

$$8 \text{ mg dexamethasone PO} = 10 \text{ mg dexamethasone sodium phosphate SC.}$$

Usual dose: 4 mg to 16 mg over 24 hours (or 5 mg to 20 mg dexamethasone sodium phosphate). Dexamethasone has a long half-life and therefore need only be given once daily, preferably in the morning. Most patients should be able to tolerate a single dose, but if CNS disturbances occur, or if high doses are involved, dexamethasone should be given in divided doses or as a continuous infusion.

Diluent: NaCl. WFI or DEX may be used.

Preparations: (as dexamethasone sodium phosphate)
UK: 5 mg/ml (2 ml)
AUS: 4 mg/ml (1 ml and 2 ml)
USA: 4 mg/ml (1 ml, 5 ml, 10 ml, 30 ml); 10 mg/ml, 20 mg/ml, 24 mg/ml (5 ml, 10 ml all)

pH: Dexamethasone is formulated as the sodium phosphate salt. This has a pH from 7–8.5.

Information: Dexamethasone has several applications in palliative care, for example:

◆ nausea and vomiting (e.g. due to refractory cases or raised intracranial pressure),

◆ raised intracranial pressure (caused by cerebral tumours, with symptoms of headache, nausea, and vomiting, blurred vision, and confusion),

- breathlessness (secondary to tumour-induced airways obstruction),
- pain (caused by nerve compression),
- anorexia/cachexia (corticosteroids stimulate appetite).

Undesirable effects include insomnia, delirium, restlessness, and myopathy. Blood glucose levels can be raised, an effect not just limited to diabetic patients. Gastroprotective drugs should be considered if an NSAID is co-prescribed; for example, if the CSCI is a short-term measure, and the oral route is unavailable, subcutaneous ranitidine may be considered, but there is no evidence to suggest that this will protect against gastroduodenal toxicity.

Dexamethasone has been reported to show concentration-dependent physical and chemical compatibility with hydromorphone and ondansetron.[30,31] Significant loss of midazolam (>10%) has been observed in some combinations of midazolam and dexamethasone stored at room temperature for 48 hours. Solutions stored at 37°C showed significant loss after 24 hours.[32] Glycopyrronium chemically interacts with dexamethasone but no precipitate forms,[33] therefore, this combination should be avoided.

Data in Chapter 4 suggest concentration-dependent incompatibility occurs with, for example, cyclizine, haloperidol, levomepromazine, and promethazine. Dexamethasone is alkaline, so it is highly likely to be incompatible with acidic solutions. See Chapter 4 for further drug compatibility data.

If dexamethasone is to be mixed with other drugs, as much diluent as possible should be added *before* the addition of dexamethasone. There may be transient turbidity with some mixtures, but a clear solution may appear soon after. If the precipitate remains, the mixture is clearly incompatible. The transient turbidity may be due to local pH changes, which causes a drug to come out of solution, or it may be due to a chemical reaction with the formation of a less soluble product. Refer to page 19 for further explanation and information about low-dose dexamethasone and site reactions.

Dexamethasone serum levels are reduced by carbamazepine, phenobarbital, and phenytoin. Higher doses will be necessary to successfully treat patients receiving these anti-epileptics.

Diamorphine

Usual dose: Providing titration occurs correctly, the dose of diamorphine can be increased, as necessary. The initial dose depends upon the patient's previous opioid treatment (see Table 2.3). A suitable starting dose for an opioid naïve patient would be 10mg diamorphine, via CSCI, over 24 hours. For patients with uncontrolled pain, the daily dose may be increased by 30–50%. Rescue doses must be available for breakthrough pain, calculated as one-sixth of the daily dose and given every 2-4 hours when necessary.

Preparations: 5 mg, 10 mg, 30 mg, 100 mg, 500 mg ampoules. This is a Schedule 2 controlled drug in the UK.

Diluent: Dilute with WFI. NaCl can also be used, up to a maximum concentration of 40 mg/ml.[34,35]

pH: 2.5–6.0. However, diamorphine is most stable within the pH range of 3.8 to 4.4 and with degradation increasing at neutral or basic pH values.[36] If diluted with NaCl, the pH must remain below 6 in order for diamorphine to remain in solution.[34]

Information: Diamorphine is a derivative of morphine. *In vivo*, following subcutaneous injection, diamorphine is rapidly absorbed and converted to the active metabolite, 6-monoacetylmorphine. This metabolite is then slowly converted to morphine.

Following oral administration, diamorphine undergoes extensive first-pass metabolism to morphine. Both diamorphine and 6-monoacetylmorphine are more lipid soluble than morphine and consequently cross the blood-brain barrier more readily. Hence, diamorphine and morphine show similar oral potencies, but different parenteral values.[37]

The major excretory products of diamorphine metabolism are morphine-3-glucuronide (M3G, the principal metabolite) and morphine-6-glucuronide (M6G). Both M6G and M3G are renally excreted. Consequently, patients in renal failure are at a greater risk of developing diamorphine (or morphine) toxicity.[38] The undesirable effects such as nausea, vomiting, drowsiness, and respiratory depression have been attributed to accumulation of M6G; undesirable effects such as myoclonus, hyperalgesia, and agitation have been attributed to accumulation of M3G.[39] However, the exact pharmacological implications of these metabolites remain unknown.

Accumulation of diamorphine metabolites can pose problems, particularly as this is likely to occur as the patient's condition deteriorates and where any signs of diamorphine toxicity may be confused with general deterioration. The use of an opioid that is not renally excreted, or is metabolized to inactive compounds would be more suitable, for example alfentanil. However, an empirical dose reduction of diamorphine between 30–50% may provide adequate analgesia, without the development of toxic effects.

Diamorphine is the opiate of choice in the UK for subcutaneous use due to its high solubility (1 g dissolves in 1.6 ml water giving final volume of 2.4 ml compared with 1 g of morphine sulphate in 21 ml of water). The initial dose depends upon the patient's current opioid requirements. Approximate opioid equivalents are shown in Table 2.3. Note that, there is great variation in the literature concerning equianalgesic doses.

Diamorphine hydrochloride and cyclizine lactate mixtures are chemically and physically stable in WFI up to concentrations of 20 mg/ml over 24 hours. If the diamorphine concentration exceeds 20 mg/ml, crystallization may occur unless the concentration of cyclizine is *no greater than* 10 mg/ml. Similarly, if the concentration of cyclizine exceeds 20 mg/ml, crystallization may occur unless the concentration of diamorphine is *no greater than* 15 mg/ml.[28]

Diamorphine has also been shown to be physically and chemically stable with various concentrations of haloperidol, hyoscine butylbromide, hyoscine hydrobromide, metoclopramide, midazolam, octreotide, and ondansetron.[29,40,41,42] Diamorphine and ketorolac mixtures in NaCl have been shown to be physically compatible.[43,44] Further drug compatibility data can be found in Chapter 4.

Diclofenac

Specialist palliative care input recommended.

Usual dose: 150 mg daily.

Diluent: NaCl. Must be given via a separate CSCI.

Preparations: 75 mg/3 ml. Not available in Australia or the USA.

pH: 7.8–9.0.

Information: *Unless benefits outweigh risks, diclofenac must not be used if there is a history of recent peptic ulceration, gastro-intestinal bleeding, or hypersensitivity to aspirin or other NSAIDs.*

Diclofenac is currently one of two NSAID drugs that may be given via a CSCI. It must be used with caution in patients with renal impairment, although this is not an absolute contra-indication in terminally ill patients. NSAIDs are often used for the treatment of bone pain. Diclofenac is also a useful analgesic for biliary or renal colic. If the oral or rectal routes are unavailable, a CSCI may be considered. However, since diclofenac can cause irritation at the site of infusion, ketorolac is often preferred. The irritation may be overcome by diluting the infusion as much as possible with NaCl. Unreported anecdotal cases suggest low-dose dexamethasone may attenuate the reaction. However, the additional risk of gastrointestinal toxicity should be considered.

When NSAIDs are administered, the prescriber must consider the need for gastroprotection and base the decision upon the presence of recognized risk factors (e.g. age greater than 65 years, previous history of peptic ulcer or bleed or concurrent usage of aspirin, warfarin, or corticosteroid).[45] Nonetheless, the risk : benefit ratio of continued NSAID use in the absence of suitable gastroprotection, must be discussed. Any dyspepsia that occurs may be successfully treated with ranitidine, via a separate CSCI; ranitidine will offer some protection, to a significantly lesser degree than proton pump inhibitors, against NSAID-induced gastroduodenal toxicity. If the risks associated with diclofenac are considered to be unacceptable, tramadol is a possible alternative and has been used successfully in the treatment of bone pain [authors' experience].

The undesirable effect profile of diclofenac is similar to other NSAIDs; the clinically important undesirable effects involve the gastrointestinal tract (ulceration; haemorrhage), and renal function (hyperkalaemia, uraemia, acute renal failure), which are more common in the elderly.

Dihydrocodeine

Specialist palliative care input recommended.

Usual dose: Providing titration occurs correctly, the dose of dihydrocodeine can be increased as necessary. However, as doses increase, the analgesic benefit may be offset by the increased incidence of undesirable effects. Dihydrocodeine is occasionally encountered, via CSCI, for use in patients with brain tumours, instead of diamorphine. Dihydrocodeine is believed to be less likely to precipitate headache, but there is no evidence to support this. Breakthrough doses are calculated as a sixth of the total daily dose, although consideration should be given to the strength of preparation available.

Preparations: 50 mg/ml. Note that parenteral dihydrocodeine is a Schedule 2 controlled drug in the UK. Unavailable in Australia and the USA.

Diluent: Dilute NaCl. WFI and DEX may also be used.

pH: 3.0–4.5.

Information: Dihydrocodeine is an analogue of codeine with weak opioid analgesic activity. Like codeine, dihydrocodeine must be metabolized to morphine for analgesia to occur; this is mediated by the cytochrome P450 system (CYP2D6 is the enzyme involved). Patients labelled as 'poor metabolizers' (CYP2D6 deficient) will not respond to dihydrocodeine. There is no recognized dose equivalence available between subcutaneous dihydrocodeine and diamorphine. Subcutaneous dihydrocodeine is approximately twice as potent as subcutaneous codeine[46] and 120 mg of intramuscular codeine is equivalent to 10 mg of intramuscular morphine.[47] Therefore, assuming that the parenteral potency applies to both subcutaneous and intramuscular routes, a conversion factor of 0.15 for subcutaneous dihydrocodeine to diamorphine appears reasonable (60 mg dihydrocodeine IM/SC = 10 mg morphine IM/SC = 6.6–10 mg diamorphine IM/SC).

Dihydrocodeine is not usually given via CSCI, although its use has been reported in certain centres. It is reported to be stable with haloperidol and midazolam.[48] Refer to Chapter 4 for further compatibility data.

Dimenhydrinate (Unavailable in the UK)

Usual dose: 50 mg to 200 mg over 24 hours. Stat doses of 25 mg to 50 mg can be given, but a dose of 400 mg should not normally be exceeded.

Diluent: NaCl, WFI, or DEX.

Preparations: 500 mg/10ml (USA)

pH: 6.4–7.2.

Information: Dimenhydrinate consists of two moieties, diphenhydramine and 8-chlorotheophylline. It is believed that the pharmacological action of dimenhydrinate results from the diphenhydramine moiety. Like cyclizine, dimenhydrinate is both an antihistaminic and antimuscarinic. The pharmacokinetics of dimenhydrinate are poorly understood. Little is known about the absorption following a subcutaneous injection, or the elimination.

It should be used with caution in patients with *closed-angle* glaucoma or paralytic ileus, due to the antimuscarinic effects. However, this is not a contra-indication for patients with advanced disease.

Dimenhydrinate is a useful antiemetic, if the cause of nausea or vomiting is due to stimulation of the vomiting centre (e.g. by radiotherapy to the head and neck, raised intracranial pressure) or vagus nerve (e.g. bowel obstruction with colic). Is also useful, if nausea and vomiting is worse on movement.

Physical and chemical compatibility has been reported with hydromorphone.[49] Dimenhydrinate is reportedly incompatible with glycopyrronium,[33] midazolam,[50] phenobarbital, and promethazine.[51] Anecdotally, it has been successfully mixed with midazolam, and a variety of other drugs, including morphine, haloperidol, metoclopramide, hyoscine butylbromide, hyoscine hydrobromide, and octreotide.[52]

The adverse effects of dimenhydrinate are a result of its pharmacology. It is sedative, which can be beneficial, although like hyoscine hydrobromide, it has the propensity to cause paradoxical agitation, usually at higher doses. Antimuscarinic effects, such as dry mouth can occur. There may also be pain at the injection/infusion site.

Fentanyl

Specialist palliative care input recommended.

Usual dose: Providing titration occurs correctly, the dose of fentanyl can be increased as necessary.

Preparations: UK: 50 micrograms/ml (2 ml, 10 ml). Schedule 2 controlled drug.

AUS: 50 micrograms/ml (2 ml, 10 ml). Schedule 8 controlled drug.

USA: 50 micrograms/ml (2 ml, 5 ml, 10 ml, 20 ml, 30 ml, 50 ml). Schedule 2 controlled drug.

Diluent: Dilute with NaCl. WFI and DEX may also be used.

pH: 4.0–7.5.

Information: Fentanyl is unlikely to be administered via a CSCI using the syringe driver because the volumes involved are too great. Alfentanil is a suitable choice, if pain control has been achieved with fentanyl and volume restricts its use. Sufentanil (not available in the UK), which is approximately 10 times more potent than fentanyl, is sometimes used when the volume of fentanyl exceeds that which can be delivered by syringe driver. There have been several case reports documenting the efficacy of fentanyl infusions in cancer patients who were unable to tolerate morphine.[8,53,54]

Fentanyl is a synthetic opioid, chemically related to pethidine, with an action primarily at the µ-receptor. It is 50–100 times more potent than morphine and approximately four times as potent as alfentanil.[55] The main route of elimination is hepatic metabolism to inactive compounds, which are mainly excreted in the urine. Co-existing liver disease should not normally necessitate a change in dose; however, an empirical dosage reduction may be required because fentanyl is extensively metabolized.

The metabolites of fentanyl are non-toxic and inactive. The use of fentanyl in patients with renal failure has not been associated with problems. Fentanyl could, therefore, be considered suitable for use in patients who are unable to tolerate diamorphine (or morphine), e.g. patients with renal failure where a dosage reduction of diamorphine does not produce the desired effect. Equianalgesic ratios are difficult to determine. However, 10 mg of morphine is stated to be approximately equivalent to 150–200 micrograms of fentanyl in patients who had previously received opioids. [8,9] Therefore, when converting from diamorphine to fentanyl, an equianalgesic factor of 0.02–0.03 should be used.

Fentanyl citrate has been shown to be stable, under stated conditions (see Chapter 4), with dexamethasone, haloperidol, hyoscine hydrobromide, ketorolac, levomepromazine, metoclopramide, midazolam, and ondansetron. [17, 56, 57]

Glycopyrronium/Glycopyrrolate

Usual dose: From 600 micrograms to 1.2 mg over 24 hours. Stat doses of 200 micrograms may be given. Doses of up to 2.4 mg have occasionally been used.

Diluent: NaCl. WFI and DEX can also be used.

Preparations: UK: 200 micrograms/ml (1 ml, 3 ml)
AUS: 200 micrograms/ml (1 ml, 2 ml)
USA: 200 micrograms/ml (1 ml, 2 ml, 5 ml, 20 ml)

pH: 2.3–4.3. The chemical stability of glycopyrronium is pH dependent. Above pH 6.0, the rate of hydrolysis increases significantly. Therefore, glycopyrronium must not be added to mixtures where the pH is above this value. Addition of an alkaline drug (e.g. phenobarbital) will more than likely produce an incompatibility.

Information: Glycopyrronium is an antimuscarinic agent with several potential uses in palliative care. As with all antimuscarinics, it should be avoided in patients with *closed-angle* glaucoma or paralytic ileus. However, this is not a contra-indication for patients with advanced disease.

Antimuscarinic drugs are used in the treatment of excessive respiratory secretions, although few trials have compared agents. One review suggested there was little difference between glycopyrronium, hyoscine butylbromide and hyoscine hydrobromide.[58] However, a recent retrospective study suggests that glycopyrronium is superior.[59] Glycopyrronium may be of benefit in the treatment of bowel colic and large-volume vomiting associated with bowel obstruction[60], possibly in combination with octreotide [authors' experience]. It may also have a role as a treatment for excessive sweating.

Glycopyrronium may be preferred to hyoscine hydrobromide for the treatment of terminal secretions for the following reasons:

(i) it is less expensive,

(ii) it does not cross the blood brain barrier so is devoid of CNS effects such as sedation and paradoxical agitation,

(iii) at normal doses, it has less of an effect on the ocular and cardiovascular systems than hyoscine hydrobromide.

Glycopyrronium does not relieve symptoms from already present
secretions. It is imperative that treatment is initiated as soon as secretions become apparent.

Adverse effects are dose-related and are associated with its pharmacology. They include dry mouth, constipation, and urinary retention. Unlike hyoscine hydrobromide, glycopyrronium can cause
tachycardia. The effect of glycopyrronium may be enhanced in renal
failure.[18]

Glycopyrronium chemically interacts with alkaline drugs. It reacts
with dexamethasone but no precipitate forms. Immediate precipitation occurs with dimenhydrinate and phenobarbital.[33] There may
also be a concentration-dependent incompatibility with cyclizine
(see Chapter 4); problems tend to occur with higher concentrations
of glycopyrronium, usually in the presence of other drugs, such as
diamorphine. Apart from these, glycopyrronium appears to be physically compatible with all other commonly used drugs. It has been shown
to be chemically and physically compatible with ondansetron.[17]
Glycopyrronium has also been shown to be physically compatible
with hydromorphone, hyoscine hydrobromide, morphine, and
promethazine.[33] See Chapter 4 for further drug compatibility data.

Since glycopyrronium is only available in a 200 micrograms/ml
concentration, the volume of injection may exceed the available syringe
volume. In such cases, a 12-hourly infusion will have to be used.

Haloperidol

Usual dose: 2.5 mg to 10 mg over 24 hours (antiemetic); 10 mg to 30 mg over 24 hours (agitation). Haloperidol has a long half life and may be given as a single bolus injection (up to doses of 10 mg).

Diluent: NaCl (although at high concentrations, approaching 2 mg/ml, precipitation has been reported to occur). WFI or DEX may also be used.

Preparations: UK: 5 mg/ml
AUS: 5 mg/ml
USA: 5 mg/ml (1 ml, 2 ml, 10 ml)

pH: 3.0–3.6.

Information: Haloperidol is an antipsychotic agent, chemically related to chlorpromazine. It is a potent dopamine D_2-receptor antagonist. Haloperidol has minimal sedative properties at the low doses employed for nausea and vomiting. Higher doses are sedative and can be used to control agitation and confusion. However, at the doses required to produce sedation, there is an increased risk of extrapyramidal reactions. Clonazepam, levomepromazine, or midazolam should be considered, if sedation is required in such a patient. Haloperidol should not be used alone in terminal restlessness if myoclonus is present, since it lowers the seizure threshold.

It is useful when nausea and vomiting is due to stimulation of the chemoreceptor trigger zone e.g. drugs (especially opioids), intestinal obstruction, or hypercalcaemia. Haloperidol can also be used to treat hiccups.

Haloperidol has been shown to be chemically and physically compatible with diamorphine.[29] It has also been shown to be physically compatible with cyclizine, hydromorphone and morphine (in DEX).[56,61,62,63] A recent study suggests that haloperidol above 1.25 mg/ml (25 mg/day in a 20 ml syringe) is incompatible with hyoscine butylbromide.[64] See Chapter 4 for further drug compatibility data.

Extrapyramidal reactions may occur in the elderly, especially if other D_2-receptor antagonists are prescribed, for example metoclopramide, levomepromazine. Fluoxetine and venlafaxine increase haloperidol serum levels and may lead to the development of extrapyramidal reactions; carbamazepine decreases serum levels.

Hydromorphone

Specialist palliative care input recommended.

Usual dose: Providing titration occurs correctly, the dose of hydromorphone can be increased as necessary. The initial dose depends upon the patient's previous opioid treatment (see Tables 2.2 and 2.4). A suitable starting dose for an opioid naïve patient would be 2 mg hydromorphone via CSCI over 24 hours. For patients with uncontrolled pain, the daily dose may be increased by 30–50%. Rescue doses must be available for breakthrough pain, calculated as one sixth of the daily dose and given every 2–4 hours when necessary.

Preparations: UK: Hydromorphone injection is currently unavailable except through 'special order' manufacturer, Martindale Pharmaceuticals Ltd in concentrations of 10 mg/ml, 20 mg/ml and 50 mg/ml. Schedule 2 controlled drug.

AUS: 2 mg/ml (1 ml); 10 mg/ml (1 ml, 5 ml, 50 ml). Schedule 8 controlled drug.

USA: 1 mg/ml, 2 mg/ml, 4 mg/ml, 10 mg/ml (1 ml, 5 ml, 20 ml all). Schedule 2 controlled drug.

Diluent: Dilute with NaCl. WFI or DEX may also be used.

pH: 4.0–5.5.

Information: Hydromorphone is a semi-synthetic derivative of morphine, with full opioid agonist properties. It is more soluble and potent than morphine and is particularly useful in countries where diamorphine is unavailable. This is ideal for CSCI, where small volumes are essential. Hydromorphone is therefore recommended for use in patients unable to tolerate morphine (outside the UK) or, in the absence of diamorphine, where large doses of morphine are involved. In the UK, it is unlikely to be encountered since three suitable opioids are already available (alfentanil, diamorphine, oxycodone).

The adverse effect profile of hydromorphone is similar to that of morphine. However, since the dose-limiting undesirable effects of morphine may be due to the accumulation of the metabolites morphine-6-glucuronide and morphine-3-glucuronide,[39] problems such as nausea, vomiting and constipation may be less severe with hydromorphone.[65]

The main metabolite is hydromorphone-3-glucuronide, which is similar in structure to the morphine equivalent and is also renally excreted. If this metabolite accumulates, for example in patients with renal failure, symptoms such as neuroexcitation or hyperalgesia would be expected to occur.[66,67,68] However, it has been suggested that hydromorphone is a safe and effective opioid in patients with renal failure.[69] Nonetheless, alfentanil remains the opioid better suited for CSCI in a patient with renal impairment.

Experience of hydromorphone administration via CSCI is mainly limited to reports from Canada and the USA.[70–73] There is great variation in the literature concerning equianalgesia with hydromorphone. The oral hydromorphone to subcutaneous hydromorphone potency ratio ranges from 2.5:1–5:1. Subcutaneous hydromorphone is stated to be 15–20 times more potent than oral morphine.[5,6] It therefore follows that the equianalgesic ratio for subcutaneous hydromorphone to morphine is 1:7.5 to 1:10 and for diamorphine 1:5 to 1:6.6.

Hydromorphone has been shown to be physically and chemically stable with dimenhydrinate[49] and dexamethasone[29] although this is concentration dependent in the latter case. Hydromorphone is chemically incompatible with hyaluronidase.[74]

Studies have shown hydromorphone to be physically stable with glycopyrronium, haloperidol, hyoscine hydrobromide, ketorolac, levomepromazine, metoclopramide, midazolam, ondansetron, and phenobarbital.[33, 56, 61, 75] See Chapter 4 for further drug compatibility data.

Hyoscine butylbromide

Not to be confused with hyoscine hydrobromide

Usual dose: 60 mg to 180 mg over 24 hours. Stat doses of 20 mg can be given.

Diluent: NaCl. WFI may also be used.

Preparations: 20 mg/ml (1 ml). Not available in the USA.

pH: 3.7–5.5.

Introduction: As for all antimuscarinic drugs, avoid in patients with closed-angle glaucoma or paralytic ileus. However, this is not a contra-indication for patients with advanced disease.

Hyoscine butylbromide is mainly used for the treatment of intestinal colic associated with bowel obstruction. It can also be used to dry terminal secretions, although it is believed to be less effective than glycopyrronium or hyoscine hydrobromide. It does not readily cross the blood brain barrier so is devoid of CNS effects such as sedation and paradoxical agitation.

Hyoscine butylbromide is also used in the treatment of large-volume vomiting that occurs with bowel obstruction.[76,77,78] It does not have a direct anti-emetic effect, but does reduce gastro-intestinal secretions. Bowel obstruction may lead to an increase in secretions, which can in turn precipitate nausea and vomiting.

Adverse effects include dry mouth, urinary retention and constipation.

Hyoscine butylbromide appears to be incompatible with cyclizine, although this reaction is concentration dependent (see Chapter 4). The combination of hyoscine butylbromide and cyclizine is often favoured for the treatment of symptoms associated with bowel obstruction. In such cases, glycopyrronium should be used instead of hyoscine butylbromide. See Chapter 4 for further drug compatibility data.

Hyoscine hydrobromide (Scopolamine hydrobromide)

Not to be confused with hyoscine butylbromide

Usual dose: 600 micrograms to 2.4 mg over 24 hours. Stat doses of 400 micrograms can be given.

Diluent: NaCl. WFI and DEX may also be used.

Preparations: UK: 400 micrograms/ml (1 ml); 600 micrograms/ml (1 ml).
AUS: 400 micrograms/ml (1 ml)
USA: 300 micrograms/ml (1 ml); 400 micrograms/ml (0.5 ml); 860 micrograms/ml (0.5 ml); 1 mg/ml (1 ml)

pH: 5.0–7.0.

Information: Hyoscine hydrobromide should be avoided in patients with closed-angle glaucoma or paralytic ileus. However, this is not a contra-indication for patients with advanced disease.

Hyoscine previously had several uses in palliative care, which included:

◆ Anti-emetic

◆ Colic associated with intestinal obstruction

◆ Bronchial secretions

◆ Sedation

Unfortunately, hyoscine hydrobromide can cause paradoxical agitation in addition to unwanted ocular and cardiovascular effects. Although the sedation provided by hyoscine hydrobromide can be beneficial, occasionally it is unwanted. For these reasons, glycopyrronium may be preferred for terminal secretions (and it may be more potent) and hyoscine butylbromide for colic. Hyoscine hydrobromide is now rarely used for its sedative or anti-emetic effects in palliative care in the UK.

Ketamine

Specialist palliative care input recommended. Use with caution in patients with intracranial hypertension

Usual dose: Starting dose usually 100 mg/day via CSCI. The dose can be increased up to 500 mg/day. Higher doses have been reported, but should be used under the supervision of a specialist.

Diluent: NaCl or DEX

Preparations: UK: 10 mg/ml (20 ml); 50 mg/ml (10 ml)
AUS: 100 mg/ml (2 ml)
USA: 10 mg/ml (20 ml); 50 mg/ml (10 ml); 100 mg/ml (5 ml)

pH: 3.5–5.5.

Information: It must be used cautiously in patients with heart disease, especially hypertension, or those at risk of raised intra-ocular pressure.

Ketamine is a general anaesthetic, but at sub-anaesthetic doses, analgesia may be obtained with minimal sedation. Larger doses have been given,[79] but there is an increased risk of undesirable effects.

It is believed to produce an analgesic effect through antagonism of the N-methyl-D-aspartate (NMDA) receptor.[80] Allodynia and hyperalgesia have been shown to be mediated via NMDA receptors. In patients who have developed these symptoms, or in patients with pain that is responding poorly to an adequate trial of opioids and common adjuvants, ketamine would be a suitable choice. *The dose of concurrent opioid must be reviewed because ketamine may restore responses to opioid analgesia, leading to opioid toxicity.*

Adverse effects include hallucinations, nightmares, confusion, delirium, tachycardia, and increased blood pressure. Haloperidol (e.g. 3 mg PO at night) or benzodiazepines (e.g. midazolam 2.5–5 mg SC PRN) have been suggested to treat the vivid dreams or nightmares.[79] There have been several case studies reporting the effectiveness of ketamine in cancer pain,[80–83] including a novel 'burst' approach (up to 500 mg via CSCI for 3–5 days).[84] A recent review of the literature concluded that there is not enough evidence to suggest ketamine improves the effectiveness of opioid treatment.[85]

Ketamine has been shown to be chemically stable with midazolam when mixed in NaCl.[86] In addition, ketamine has been shown to be physically stable when mixed with morphine.[87] Refer to Chapter 4 for further compatibility data.

Note that ketamine is only available in the UK for use in Primary Care on a named patient basis. The doctor completes a prescription as usual, but the pharmacist should contact the manufacturer or wholesaler to initiate supply.

Ketorolac

Specialist palliative care input recommended.

Usual dose: 30 mg to 120 mg over 24 hours.

Diluent: NaCl or DEX. WFI can be used.

Preparations: UK: 10 mg/ml (1 ml), 30 mg/ml (1 ml)
AUS: 10 mg/ml (1 ml), 30 mg/ml (1 ml)
USA: 15 mg/ml, 30 mg/ml (1 ml, 2 ml, 10 ml all)

pH: 7.0–8.0.

Information: Unless benefits outweigh risks, ketorolac must not be used if there is a history of recent peptic ulceration, gastro-intestinal bleeding, or hypersensitivity to aspirin or other NSAIDs.

Ketorolac must be used with **extreme caution** in patients with moderate-severe renal failure, or patients at risk of haemorrhage or incomplete haemostasis (e.g. liver disease).

Ketorolac is a NSAID with strong analgesic activity. It should only be used for bone pain where other NSAID formulations (e.g. diclofenac suppositories) are impractical or ineffective. Note that oral ketorolac has a direct irritant effect on the gastric mucosa in addition to the systemic effect. Therefore, subcutaneous ketorolac may be preferred. *Concurrent opioid dose reduction should be considered and other NSAIDs (if any) must be discontinued.*

There are no clinical trials to date involving the use of subcutaneous ketorolac in palliative care, only case studies.[43,88,89] A proton pump inhibitor **must** be co-prescribed as prophylaxis against peptic ulceration. If oral treatment is impossible, the use of ketorolac must be reviewed. However, the risk:benefit ratio of using of ketorolac in the terminal stages of life without gastroprotective drugs would appear to be acceptable.

Although ranitidine is physically compatible with ketorolac (see Chapter 4), it will only offer a degree of protection, significantly less than a proton pump inhibitor, against NSAID-induced gastroduodenal toxicity. Ranitidine will, however, treat the dyspepsia that may occur with ketorolac. If the risks associated with ketorolac are considered to be unacceptable, tramadol has been used successfully in the treatment of bone pain [authors' experience].

The undesirable effect profile of ketorolac is similar to other NSAIDs; the clinically important undesirable effects involve the gastro-intestinal tract (ulceration; haemorrhage) and renal function (hyperkalaemia, uraemia, acute renal failure) which are more common in the elderly. Regular checks on renal function should be performed (if clinically indicated) because ketorolac-induced renal toxicity is associated with increasing levels of serum creatinine and potassium.[90]

Ketorolac has been shown to be physically stable in NaCl with diamorphine, dependent upon concentrations.[43,44] It is unlikely to be compatible with most drugs given in the syringe driver due to the alkaline pH, although as shown in Chapter 4, it is physically compatible with ranitidine.

Levomepromazine (Methotrimeprazine)

Usual dose: 6.25 mg to 25 mg over 24 hours (antiemetic); 25 mg to 200 mg over 24 hours for agitation. Irritation is possible at the infusion site. For lower doses, a bolus subcutaneous injection can be given to overcome the problem. This is usually given at night. If an infusion is still required, and irritation becomes a problem, refer to page 17 for the management of site reactions.

Diluent: NaCl. WFI and DEX have also been used.

Preparations: 25 mg/ml (1 ml). Available through the SAS scheme only in Australia (see Appendix 2). Unavailable in the USA.

pH: 4.5.

Information: Levomepromazine is a broad spectrum antiemetic with a strong sedative effect. Note that a subcutaneous dose is believed to be twice as potent as that administered orally (i.e. 6.25 mg SC = 12.5 mg PO). It acts on the main receptor sites involved in the vomiting pathway (dopamine D_2-receptors, serotonin 5-HT_2-receptors, histamine H_1-receptors and acetylcholine muscarinic receptors).

Doses above 50 mg/24 hours should be used cautiously in ambulatory patients because of the problems of sedation and postural hypotension. It is used at low doses to treat intractable nausea and vomiting. Levomepromazine has a long half life and can be given as a single daily dose at night to avoid the problems of sedation.[91] At higher doses, it is a powerful sedative and can be used to treat terminal restlessness. However, if myoclonus is present, a benzodiazepine would be a more suitable choice, or should at least be included in the treatment regimen.

Levomepromazine displays concentration-dependent incompatibility when mixed with dexamethasone. Solutions containing levomepromazine have developed a purple discolouration in UV light and should be discarded.[92] Levomepromazine has been shown to be physically compatible with methadone, morphine sulphate, hydromorphone and fentanyl.[26] It has been reported to be incompatible with ranitidine,[125] although data in Chapter 4 suggest a concentration-dependent incompatibility. Refer to Chapter 4 for further compatibility data.

Undesirable effects include sedation, postural hypotension, dry mouth, and extrapyramidal reactions (especially if other D_2-receptor antagonists are given). Hallucinations may occur rarely. Levomepromazine antagonizes the treatment of Parkinson's disease.

Methadone

To be initiated only in specialist palliative care centres

Usual dose: Provided titration occurs correctly, the dose of methadone can be increased as necessary. A CSCI must not be started in a methadone naïve patient, unless under expert supervision. The initial dose depends upon the patient's previous oral methadone dose. Providing the patient has been successfully titrated with oral methadone, the total daily subcutaneous dose is estimated to be *50%* of the oral.[93] This can be given as a CSCI. Rescue doses for breakthrough pain are calculated as *one sixth* of the total daily dose and are given *no more frequently than every three hours.* If two or more rescue doses are required, the total daily dose should be increased by 30%.

Preparations: UK: 10 mg/ml (1 ml, 2 ml, 3.5 ml, 5 ml). Schedule 2 controlled drug.
AUS: 10 mg/ml (1 ml). Schedule 8 controlled drug.
USA: 10 mg/ml (20 ml). Schedule 2 controlled drug.

Diluent: Methadone should be diluted maximally in the syringe with NaCl. WFI, or DEX can also be used.

pH: 4.5–7.0.

Information: Methadone is a synthetic opioid agonist with greater affinity than morphine for both δ- and μ-receptors. In addition, methadone exhibits non-competitive N-methyl-D-aspartate (NMDA) antagonist activity that may explain its suggested benefit in neuropathic pain.[93] It is readily absorbed following subcutaneous injection and is metabolized in the liver to inactive compounds that are excreted in bile and urine.

Hepatic impairment does not unduly affect methadone metabolism and dosage adjustments should not be necessary in stable disease states, although acute changes in hepatic function will require dosage adjustments. Dosage adjustments are not required for patients in renal failure, which allows methadone to be a suitable choice for use in patients who are unable to tolerate morphine.

Methadone has a high bio-availability and very long elimination half-life of over thirty hours. This extremely long half-life shows wide interpatient variation and accumulation can occur with continuous use. Consequently, the dose of methadone is highly individualized.[94] Methadone can cause severe irritation at the site of the infusion. Several methods for overcoming this problem have been suggested.[95,96] However, the following is recommended (see also page 17):

◆ Usual diluent is NaCl; DEX is occasionally used. WFI is unlikely to improve the tolerability of the infusion site.

◆ Rotate the site every 2 days.

◆ Hyaluronidase is occasionally used, although there is no direct evidence to support its use. It is recommended that a dose of 150 units per site is used in patients experiencing local toxicity with methadone. Hyaluronidase must not be added to the syringe because it degrades over the 24-hour infusion period. It is injected directly into the site, prior to the infusion, via the butterfly needle and giving set; it should not be injected directly into an inflamed site.

◆ Some centres both in the UK and abroad recommend the use of 1 mg dexamethasone to be added to the syringe.[95,96] This appears to attenuate local toxicity and the mixture appears to be physically stable (since expected clinical outcome is observed). However, if other drugs are to be added to the syringe (such as glycopyrronium), dexamethasone can cause compatibility problems. In this case, inject the dexamethasone directly into the infusion site and flush with a small volume of NaCl (e.g. 0.5 ml).

Methadone has been shown to be physically compatible with dexamethasone, haloperidol, hyoscine butylbromide, ketorolac, levomepromazine, metoclopramide and midazolam.[26]

Carbamazepine, phenobarbital, phenytoin, and rifampicin may reduce the effect of methadone; cimetidine, fluoxetine, and monoamine oxidase inhibitors may increase the toxicity of methadone, so concomitant use should be avoided. Methadone may increase zidovudine levels.

Metoclopramide

Usual dose: 30 to 120 mg over 24 hours.

Diluent: NaCl. WFI and DEX can also be used.

Preparations: UK: 5 mg/ml (2 ml)

AUS: 5 mg/ml (2 ml)

USA: 5 mg/ml (2 ml, 10 ml, 20 ml, 30 ml)

pH: 3.0–5.0.

Information: Must not be used if complete intestinal obstruction is present or suspected.

Metoclopramide is a D_2-receptor antagonist, with non-sedating antiemetic and prokinetic properties. It is useful in the treatment of nausea and vomiting caused by drugs, gastric stasis, or partial outflow obstruction. The inclusion of dexamethasone to the regimen in the latter two cases can improve the treatment of nausea and vomiting.

Extrapyramidal reactions can occur with metoclopramide, especially if other D_2-receptor antagonists (e.g. haloperidol, levomepromazine) are used. These reactions are more common in young females, or the elderly. Doses of up to 60 mg are used regularly in palliative care and such reactions have rarely occurred. Metoclopramide antagonizes the treatment of Parkinson's disease.

Dosage reductions of up to 50% may be necessary in patients with moderate to severe renal impairment. An empirical dosage reduction may be necessary in patients with a significant degree of hepatic impairment. $5-HT_3$ antagonists and antimuscarinic drugs can directly interfere with the prokinetic action. For example, when used with cyclizine, dimenhydrinate, hyoscine, or ondansetron, higher doses of metoclopramide may be required to achieve the desired prokinetic effect. Metoclopramide can cause irritation at the site of injection. Due to the presence of chloride ions in the injection formulation, crystallization *may* occur with cyclizine. The solution should be discarded if it discolours. Metoclopramide has been shown to be physically and chemically compatible with diamorphine.[29]

In addition, it has been shown to be physically compatible with fentanyl, hydromorphone, methadone, and morphine.[56] See Chapter 4 for further drug compatibility data.

Midazolam

Usual dose: 10mg to 60mg over 24 hours for seizures, anxiety, or terminal agitation. If agitation is poorly controlled at this maximum dose, the additional use of levomepromazine should be considered. Clonazepam or phenobarbital may be considered for control of seizures.

Diluent: NaCl. WFI and DEX may also be used.

Preparations: UK: 5 mg/ml (2 ml)

AUS: 1 mg/ml (5 ml), 5 mg/ml (1 ml, 3 ml, 10 ml)

USA: 1 mg/ml, 5 mg/ml (1 ml, 2 ml, 5 ml, 10 ml all)

pH: 2.9–3.7.

Information: Midazolam is a short-acting benzodiazepine, which is suitable for CSCI. It is metabolized in the liver mainly to a less active metabolite which is excreted in the urine. Empirical dosage reductions may be necessary in liver disease (main site of metabolism) and renal disease (accumulation of metabolite).

Like clonazepam, midazolam has several uses in palliative care:

+ Terminal agitation
+ Myoclonus
+ Seizures
+ Intractable hiccup
+ Anxiety

Unlike clonazepam, midazolam has not been shown to be of benefit in neuropathic pain. Midazolam is preferred to clonazepam in emergency situations, such as major haemorrhage, because of its quicker onset of action. Although indicated for the treatment of hiccups, midazolam has been implicated as a cause of drug-induced hiccups.[97]

Midazolam has been shown to be physically and chemically compatible with alfentanil,[16] diamorphine,[40] and ondansetron.[17] It is incompatible with dimenhydrinate[50] and ranitidine.[98] Significant loss of midazolam has been observed in some combinations of midazolam and dexamethasone, particularly when solution is stored at 37° C.[34] Finally, midazolam has been shown to be physically compatible with fentanyl, hydromorphone, methadone and morphine.[56] Tolerance has been reported to develop rapidly (within a week) to the effects of midazolam, requiring increasing doses, or the introduction of another drug.[99]

Morphine

Usual dose: There is no maximum dose of morphine in palliative care. A suitable starting dose in an opioid naïve patient would be 10–20 mg daily, via syringe driver. If pain is uncontrolled, the dose can be increased by 30–50%. Rescue doses must be available for breakthrough pain and are calculated as one sixth of the total daily dose.

Preparations:

Morphine sulphate:

UK: 10 mg/ml, 15 mg/ml, 20 mg/ml, 30 mg/ml (1 ml, 2 ml all). Schedule 2 controlled drug.

AUS: 5 mg/ml, 10 mg/ml, 15 mg/ml, 30 mg/ml (1 ml all). Schedule 8 controlled drug.

USA: 0.5 mg/ml (2 ml, 10 ml), 1 mg/ml (2 ml, 30 ml, 60 ml), 2 mg/ml (1 ml, 30 ml), 4 mg/ml (1 ml, 2 ml), 5 mg/ml (1 ml, 30 ml), 8 mg/ml (1 ml), 10 mg/ml (1 ml, 2 ml, 10 ml, 30 ml), 15 mg/ml (1 ml, 20 ml), 25 mg/ml (1 ml, 10 ml, 20 ml, 30 ml, 40 ml, 50 ml), 50 mg/ml (10 ml, 20 ml, 30 ml, 50 ml). Schedule 2 controlled drug.

Morphine tartrate: 120 mg/1.5 ml, 400 mg/5 ml (AUS). Schedule 8 controlled drug.

Morphine hydrochloride: various formulations available (not UK, AUS or USA)

Diluent: Dilute with NaCl, or DEX. WFI may also be used.

pH: 2.5–6.5. As with diamorphine, degradation increases at neutral or basic pH values.

Information: Orally, it is the opiate of choice for the treatment of moderate-severe cancer pain. Morphine is not widely administered in the UK via CSCI because of the availability of diamorphine. Nevertheless, where problems with supply of diamorphine exist, morphine sulphate is an acceptable alternative. Morphine is used extensively around of the world. Use of morphine tartrate overcomes the volume limitations encountered with the hydrochloride and sulphate salts for use in syringe drivers. The limits of solubility of the morphine salts differ and are as follows: hydrochloride 1 part in 24 parts water; sulphate 1 part in 21 parts of water; tartrate 1 part in 10 parts of water. Pharmacokinetic and compatibility information is the same as for morphine sulphate.

After subcutaneous injection, morphine is well absorbed and is predominantly metabolized in the liver to morphine-3-glucuronide (M3G, the principal metabolite) and morphine-6-glucuronide (M6G). The actual clinical implications of M6G and M3G are yet to be elucidated. However, it is believed that M6G is pharmacologically active and is more potent than morphine at the μ-receptor.[39] The major metabolite, M3G, is apparently devoid of analgesic activity and it has been suggested that it may actually antagonize the analgesic efficacy of morphine.[100]

Both M6G and M3G are renally excreted. Consequently, patients in renal failure are at a greater risk of developing morphine toxicity.[38] The undesirable effects such as nausea, vomiting, drowsiness, and respiratory depression have been attributed to accumulation of M6G; undesirable effects such as myoclonus, hyperalgesia, and agitation have been attributed to accumulation of M3G.[39]

Accumulation of morphine metabolites can pose problems, particularly as this is likely to occur as the patient's condition deteriorates and where any signs of morphine toxicity may be confused with general deterioration. The use of an opioid that is not renally excreted, or is metabolized to inactive compounds would be more suitable, for example alfentanil. However, an empirical dose reduction of morphine between 30–50% may provide adequate analgesia, without the development of toxic effects.

Subcutaneous morphine is considered to be 2–3 times as potent as oral morphine.[5,6,101] A range is stated because much of the analgesic activity of morphine is believed to be due to production of M6G,[102] a factor that varies between patients. Intravenous morphine is considered to be equipotent to subcutaneous morphine.[103] When converting from oral morphine to subcutaneous diamorphine, a ratio of 3:1 is commonly used.[1] The equianalgesic ratio for subcutaneous diamorphine to subcutaneous morphine is difficult to predict from the literature. Values suggested range from 1 : 1 to 3 : 2 (refer to Table 2.2).

Morphine sulphate has been shown to be chemically and physically compatible with hyoscine hydrobromide, metoclopramide, midazolam, and ondansetron.[17,29,40,75] Morphine sulphate has also been shown to be physically compatible with clonazepam, dexamethasone, dimenhydrinate, glycopyrronium, haloperidol (diluted with dextrose 5%), hyoscine butylbromide, ketamine, ketorolac, levomepromazine, promethazine, and ranitidine.[23,33,56,63,104,105] See Chapter 4 for further drug compatibility data.

Octreotide

Specialist palliative care input recommended.

Usual dose: 300 micrograms to 600 micrograms over 24 hours.

Diluent: NaCl is the recommended diluent. WFI or DEX can also be used.

Preparations: UK: 50 micrograms/ml, 100 micrograms/ml and 500 micrograms/ml (1 ml all); 200 micrograms/ml (5 ml)

AUS: 50 micrograms/ml, 100 micrograms/ml and 500 micrograms/ml (1 ml all)

USA: 50 micrograms/ml, 100 micrograms/ml, 200 micrograms/ml, 500 micrograms/ml, 1 micrograms/ml (1.5 ml all)

pH: 3.9–4.5.

Information: Octreotide is a somatostatin analogue that has potentially several roles in palliative care. One of its actions involves reduction of intestinal secretions of water and sodium, in addition to stimulating absorption of water and electrolytes. It is therefore useful in situations where excessive diarrhoea (e.g. carcinoid syndrome) or large-volume vomiting is present.

Octreotide has an as yet undefined role in the management of gastrointestinal obstruction. It is an expensive drug and should not be used routinely to treat this condition; patients prescribed octreotide should be regularly reviewed and drug treatment stopped if there is no clear benefit. There have been several case reports of the effectiveness of octreotide,[75,106–108] and several small controlled trials[76,109,110] that clearly show the benefit of octreotide in relieving symptoms. Doses above 600 micrograms are not thought to improve symptom control further,[111] although some centres use over 1000 micrograms. Combination with an antimuscarinic drug such as hyoscine butylbromide[78] or glycopyrronium [authors' experience] may further improve symptom control.

In the absence of stability data it would be wise to administer octreotide either as a separate CSCI, or as a bolus subcutaneous injection. In the latter case, the ampoule should be warmed prior to injection, to reduce pain on administration.

Octreotide has been shown to be physically and chemically compatible with diamorphine.[41] Refer to Chapter 4 for further drug compatibility data.

Undesirable effects include dry mouth (although tolerance should develop) and flatulence (reduce dose and increase slowly).

Ondansetron

Specialist palliative care input recommended.

Usual dose: 24 mg over 24 hours. Up to 32 mg may be given. Maximum 8 mg in severe hepatic disease.

Diluent: NaCl. WFI and DEX can also be used.

Preparations: UK: 2 mg/ml (2 ml, 4 ml)
AUS: 2 mg/ml (2 ml, 4 ml)
USA: 2 mg/ml (2 ml, 20 ml); 32 mg/50 ml

pH: 3.3–4.0. Ondansetron may precipitate with alkaline drugs.

Information: It is a selective 5-HT$_3$ antagonist with proven efficacy in the treatment of acute nausea and vomiting associated with radiotherapy to the upper abdomen, and chemotherapy. The place of ondansetron in palliative medicine remains to be determined. There have been case reports [112,113] stating good results in patients unresponsive to conventional anti-emetic treatment. In addition, ondansetron has been shown to be beneficial in patients with pruritus associated with a variety of causes.[114–117] The main adverse effect is constipation. Consequently, ondansetron may be of benefit in treating the diarrhoea associated with carcinoid syndrome.

Serotonin is released by enterochromaffin cells in the bowel wall in response to certain stimuli, in particular bowel distension. It is also implicated in the nausea and vomiting associated with renal failure.

Ondansetron may be a suitable second or third line treatment in patients with such conditions who have failed to respond to conventional anti-emetics. The dose should be reduced in liver disease, with a maximum dose of 8 mg in severe hepatic impairment.

There is limited stability data available, but ondansetron is compatible with diamorphine (in NaCl) at concentrations up to 0.64 mg/ml and 5 mg/ml respectively.[42] Studies have shown ondansetron to be physically and chemically compatible with alfentanil, dexamethasone (higher concentrations likely to be incompatible), fentanyl, glycopyrronium, midazolam, metoclopramide, and morphine sulphate.[17,31]

Ondansetron may interfere with the analgesic effect of tramadol; serotonin is one of the main neurotansmitters implicated in the down modulation of spinal nociception and antagonism of spinal 5-HT$_3$ receptors by ondansetron has been shown to reduce the analgesic efficacy of tramadol.[118]

Oxycodone

Specialist palliative care input recommended.

Usual dose: There is no maximum dose of oxycodone in palliative care. The initial dose depends upon the patient's previous opioid treatment (see Table 2.2 for equianalgesic ratios). For opioid naive patients, a suitable starting dose would be 5–10 mg over 24 hours. If pain is uncontrolled, this dose can be increased by 30–50%. Rescue doses should be given for breakthrough pain and are calculated as one sixth of the total daily opioid dose.

Preparations: 10 mg/ml, 20 mg/2 ml [UK]. Schedule 2 controlled drug.

Diluent: Dilute with NaCl. WFI or DEX may also be used.

pH: 4.5–5.5.

Information: Oxycodone is a semi-synthetic opioid with similar properties to morphine. Unlike morphine, oxycodone only displays weak μ-receptor binding affinity; analgesia is believed to be due to the high affinity binding to κ-receptors.[119]

Oxycodone is a suitable alternative to either diamorphine or alfentanil. Although its place in therapy is currently unclear it would seem appropriate to consider oxycodone injection as a first line option for patients previously controlled with oral oxycodone. Refer to Table 2.2 for equianalgesic ratios. The manufacturer states that subcutaneous oxycodone is equivalent in potency to subcutaneous diamorphine; in addition, 2 mg of oral oxycodone is stated to be equivalent to 1 mg of subcutaneous oxycodone.[7] These statements are not in agreement with current beliefs (60 mg oral morphine = 20 mg subcutaneous diamorphine; 60 mg oral morphine = 30 mg oral oxycodone = 15 mg parenteral oxycodone); however, it must be emphasized that equianalgesic ratios serve only as a guide.

Oxycodone is well absorbed after subcutaneous administration. Intravenous, intramuscular, and subcutaneous administration of oxycodone are considered to be bioequivalent.[7] Oxycodone is metabolized to noroxycodone (considered to be inactive) and, to a lesser extent, oxymorphone (although more potent than morphine, oxymorphone is unlikely to produce a significant effect[120,121]). The manufacturer states that oxycodone is contra-indicated in hepatic impairment, presumably because oxycodone concentrations increase. In renal impairment, although there are no significant metabolites as with morphine, oxycodone plasma concentrations may increase by up to 50%.[122,123] Therefore, empirical dosage reductions may be necessary should oxycodone be used in patients with hepatic and/or renal impairment.

Oxycodone has been shown to be chemically and physically compatible with dexamethasone sodium phosphate, haloperidol, hyoscine butylbromide, hyoscine hydrobromide, levomepromazine, metoclopramide and midazolam.[124] Oxycodone has been shown to be physically compatible with cyclizine, ketamine, ketorolac, octreotide, ondansetron and ranitidine, in addition to multiple drug combinations.[125] Note that oxycodone and cyclizine combinations display concentration-dependent incompatibility. See Chapter 4 for further compatibility information.

Phenobarbital (Phenobarbitone)

Specialist palliative care input recommended.

Usual dose: 200 mg to 600 mg over 24 hours. Higher doses up to 2400 mg have been used. Subcutaneous bolus doses are painful and should be avoided. If necessary, between 50 mg to 200 mg may be given as a bolus dose via IM or IV injection.

Diluent: WFI, or NaCl.

Preparations: UK: 30 mg/ml,   60 mg/ml,   200 mg/ml   (1 ml   all).
Schedule 3 controlled drug.
AUS: 40 mg/ml (0.5 ml); 200 mg/ml (1 ml)
USA: 30 mg/ml, 60 mg/ml, 65 mg/ml, 130 mg/ml
(1 ml all)

pH: 10.0–11.0. Subcutaneous bolus injections can cause tissue necrosis due to the high pH. However, a CSCI is usually well tolerated.

Information: Phenobarbital is a long-acting barbiturate. It may be useful in palliative care as an anti-epileptic. If a patient is unable to take oral anticonvulsants, and a benzodiazepine is ineffective or impractical, phenobarbital can be given for epilepsy prophylaxis/ treatment. In addition, phenobarbital can be given to treat refractory terminal restlessness.[126]

It is formulated at an alkaline pH and is therefore unlikely to be stable with most drugs. It should therefore be given via separate CSCI.

Promethazine

Specialist palliative care input recommended.

Usual dose: 50–150 mg over 24 hours. Stat doses of 25 mg to 50 mg can be given.

Diluent: NaCl. WFI, or DEX can also be used.

Preparations: UK: 25 mg/ml (1 ml, 2 ml)
AUS: 25 mg/ml (2 ml)
USA: 25 mg/ml (1 ml), 50 mg/ml (1 ml)

pH: 4.0–5.5. Likely to be incompatible with alkaline drugs.

Information: Promethazine is a useful drug, having antihistaminic, antimuscarinic and antidopaminergic properties. These pharmacological actions confer useful anti-emetic and sedative properties. It is metabolized in the liver to inactive promethazine sulphoxide and glucuronides. Promethazine should be used with caution in patients with glaucoma or paralytic ileus, although this is not a contra-indication for patients with advanced disease.

Promethazine can be used an anti-emetic if the cause of nausea or vomiting is due to stimulation of the vomiting centre (e.g. by radio-therapy to the head and neck, raised intracranial pressure), vagus nerve (e.g. bowel obstruction with colic), chemoreceptor trigger zone (e.g. drugs, hypercalcaemia, bowel obstruction) or is worse on movement.

Promethazine is incompatible with dimenhydrinate (although there should be no need to co-prescribe these drugs).[51] It is also incompatible with ketorolac.[127] Promethazine has been shown to be physically compatible with glycopyrronium.[33] Anecdotally, it has been reported to mix with morphine sulphate and precipitate with midazolam.[128]

The main undesirable effects of promethazine are related to its pharmacology. It is sedative, which can be beneficial, although like hyoscine hydrobromide, it has the propensity to cause paradoxical agitation, usually at higher doses. Antimuscarinic effects, such as dry mouth can occur. Extrapyramidal reactions can also occur; again these may occur at higher doses. Sterile abscesses or necrotic lesions have been reported on rare occasions following subcutaneous use of promethazine. However, anecdotal evidence[128] suggests that a CSCI of promethazine is both effective and well tolerated and the use of low-dose dexamethasone (see page 19) appears to increase the tolerability of a CSCI.[129]

Ranitidine

Specialist palliative care input recommended.

Usual dose: 150 mg to 300 mg over 24 hours

Preparations: UK: 25 mg/ml (2 ml)
AUS: 25 mg/ml (2 ml)
USA: 0.5 mg/ml, 25 mg/ml (2 ml, 10 ml, 40 ml all)

Diluent: NaCl. WFI and DEX can also be used.

pH: 6.7–7.3.

Information: The H_2 antagonists reduce both gastric acid output and the volume of gastric secretions. Although not as effective as the proton pump inhibitors, ranitidine may afford some protection against NSAID-induced peptic ulceration and reduce the symptoms of dyspepsia that may occur. Ranitidine can be infused concurrently with ketorolac (see Chapter 4). Note, however, there is no evidence to suggest that a CSCI of ranitidine will prevent NSAID-induced gastroduodenal damage.

Ranitidine is incompatible with midazolam and phenobarbital.[98,130] It has been reported to be incompatible with levomepromazine,[125] although data in Chapter 4 suggest a concentration-dependent incompatibility. Refer to Chapter 4 for further compatibility data.

Sufentanil

Specialist palliative care input recommended.

Usual dose: There is no maximum dose of sufentanil. The initial dose depends upon the patient's previous opioid treatment. In general, sufentanil is only used in patients receiving fentanyl when the volume required to administer fentanyl exceeds the volume allowable in the syringe driver. Alfentanil is another alternative to fentanyl.

Preparations: UK: Not available

AUS: Sufentanil citrate 375 micrograms/5 ml (equivalent to Sufentanil 250 micrograms/ml). Available only through SAS scheme. Schedule 8 controlled drug.

USA: 50 micrograms/ml (1 ml, 2 ml, 5 ml). Schedule 2 controlled drug.

Diluent: NaCl. WFI and DEX may also be used

pH: 4.5–7.0.

Information: Sufentanil is a highly potent opioid analgesic. It is about 7–10 times more potent than fentanyl in man.[8] Major sites of biotransformation are the liver and kidney, where it is metabolized by N-dealkylation and O-demethylation. The metabolites are excreted in the urine. About 2% of the dose is eliminated as unchanged drug. Sufentanil is extensively bound to plasma proteins (>90%). The terminal elimination half-life of sufentanil is about 2.5 hours.

Tramadol

Specialist palliative care input recommended.

Usual dose: 100 to 600 mg over 24 hours; doses above 600 mg are not recommended. Although breakthrough doses are calculated as one sixth of the total daily dose, the use of PRN tramadol doses of 50–100 mg SC should *initially* be avoided due to the high risk of undesirable effects, such as nausea. If tramadol is to be added to a treatment regime, 100 mg via CSCI is an appropriate starting dose, with 25–50 mg PRN for breakthrough pain.

Preparations: 50 mg/ml (2 ml). Is a Schedule 4 drug in Australia. Not available in the USA.

Diluent: NaCl. WFI and DEX may also be used.

pH: 6.0–6.8.

Information: Tramadol is a centrally acting synthetic compound which is structurally related to codeine. Its efficacy is believed to fit between codeine and morphine. Tramadol produces its analgesic effect through two distinct, yet synergistic, pharmacological mechanisms. It is a racemic mixture, the two enantiomers (mirror images) having distinct pharmacological profiles. The (+) enantiomer binds weakly to the µ-receptor, with an affinity 10 times less than codeine. The (+) enantiomer also inhibits neuronal reuptake of serotonin. The (−) enantiomer is believed to inhibit neuronal reuptake of noradrenaline (norepinephrine) only. The analgesic effect of racemic tramadol is greater than the sum of its parts, suggesting that the two enantiomers act synergistically.[131] The only active metabolite of tramadol, (+)-O-desmethyltramadol, (M1), has a higher affinity for the µ-receptor than (+)-tramadol itself. The analgesia produced by tramadol is only partially reduced by naloxone and almost completely reversed by the α_2 antagonist, yohimbine.[132,133] This suggests that tramadol achieves analgesia through the synergy of spinal modulation of pain via activation of postsynaptic α_2 receptors and its weak opioid activity.

Elimination is primarily by hepatic cytochrome P450 mediated metabolism (CYP2D6 is the enzyme responsible for the production of M1) whilst up to 30% is excreted by the kidneys unchanged. The majority of the metabolites are also excreted by the kidneys. Consequently, enzyme inducers (e.g. carbamazepine) or inhibitors (e.g. quinidine for CYP2D6) of drug metabolism will modify the elimination of tramadol. Patients labelled as 'poor metabolizers' (CYP2D6 deficient) will have a reduced response to tramadol but nonetheless will achieve analgesia (see dihydrocodeine). If renal function is moderately impaired, or hepatic function is severely impaired, an empirical dosage reduction will be necessary (e.g. 30–50%, dependent upon response).

Tramadol is rarely administered via CSCI. Occasionally, however, a patient may have obtained benefit from oral administration, or the patient may not be able to tolerate NSAIDs. Tramadol also appears to be of benefit in neuropathic pain.[134] It is in these situations that tramadol via CSCI could be considered. Since tramadol is only a weak opioid, there is no reason why it cannot be combined with a strong opioid, such as diamorphine, with the potential of even greater synergy. Tramadol has indeed been combined with morphine with good effect, with the observation that the dose of the strong opioid could be reduced.[136]

Equianalgesic ratios between subcutaneous tramadol and diamorphine do not exist and are difficult to predict since the pharmacology of tramadol is multimodal (see above). Nonetheless, parenteral tramadol is stated to be approximately one eighth to one tenth as potent as parenteral morphine.[62,64] Based on the conversion range of subcutaneous diamorphine:morphine of 1 : 1 to 3 : 2, a conversion ratio for tramadol:diamorphine of 12 : 1 is suggested.

Undesirable effects, especially nausea, are dose-dependent and therefore more likely to appear with higher doses. The use of a CSCI will reduce the initial peak plasma concentration and should, in theory, reduce the incidence of such effects. Initial treatment with 100 mg PRN doses should be avoided in order to improve patient acceptance. If the decision to use tramadol is made, a suitable starting dose of 100 mg via CSCI is acceptable. Other undesirable effects are generally similar to those of opioids, although they are usually less severe.

Ondansetron may interfere with the analgesic effect of tramadol; serotonin is one of the main neurotansmitters implicated in the down modulation of spinal nociception and antagonism of spinal 5-HT$_3$ receptors by ondansetron has been shown to reduce the analgesic efficacy of tramadol.[118]

References

1. Regnard CFB, Tempest S. *A Guide to Symptom Relief in Advanced Cancer*. 4th edn. Hochland & Hochland Ltd. Hale;1998.

2. Cherry NI. Opioid Analgesics. Comparative Features and Prescribing Guidelines. *Drugs* 1996; **51**(5):713–737.

3. Kirkham SR, Pugh R. Opioid analgesia in uraemic patients. *Lancet* 1995; **345**:1185.

4. Doyle D, Hanks GWC, Cherney N, Calman K (eds). *Oxford Textbook of Palliative Medicine*. 3rd edn. Oxford University Press Oxford; 2003.

5. Levy MH. Pharmacologic treatment of cancer pain. *N Engl J Med* 1996; **335**(15):1124–1132.

6. Lothian ST, Fotis MA, Von Gunten CF, Lyons J *et al*. Cancer pain management through a pharmacist-based analgesic dosing service. *Am J Health-Syst Pharm* 1999; **56**:1119–1125.

7. Data on file. Napp Pharmaceuticals Ltd. 2004.

8. Paix A, Coleman A, Lees J , Grigson J *et al*. Subcutaneous fentanyl and sufentanil infusion substitution for morphine intolerance in cancer pain management. *Pain* 1995; **63**:263–269.

9. Hunt R, Fazekas B, Thorne D, Brooksbank M. A Comparison of Subcutaneous Morphine and Fentanyl in Hospice Cancer Patients. *J Pain Symptom Manage* 1999; **18**:111–119.

10. Silvasti M, Svartling N, Pitkanen M, Rosenberg PH. Comparison of intravenous patient controlled analgesia with tramadol versus morphine after microvascular breast reconstruction. *Eur J Anaesthesiol* 2000; **17**:448–455.

11. Larijani GE, Goldberg ME. Alfentanil hydrochloride: A new short acting narcotic analgesic for surgical procedures. *Clin Pharm* 1987; **6**:275–282.

12. Tegeder I, Lotsch J, Geisslinger G. Pharmacokinetics of opioids in liver disease. *Clin Pharmacokinet* 1999; **37**:17–40.

13. Maitre PO, Vozeh S, Heykants J *et al*. Population pharmacokinetics of alfentanil: the average dose-plasma concentration relationship and interindividual variability in patients. *Anaesthesiology* 1987; **66**:3–12.

14. Hill HF, Coda BA, Mackie AM, Iverson K. Patient controlled analgesic infusions: alfentanil versus morphine. *Pain* 1992; **49**:301–310.

15. Schragg S, Checketts MR, Kenny GN. Lack of rapid development of opioid toxicity during alfentanil and remifentanil infusions for post-operative pain. *Anesth Analg* 1999; **89**:753–757.

16. Mehta AC, Kay EA. Storage time can now be extended. *Pharm Pract* 1997; **7**:305–308.

17. Stewart JT, Warren FW, King DT, Venkateshwaran TG *et al*. Stability of ondansetron hydrochloride and 12 medications in plastic syringes. *Am J Health Syst Pharm* 1998; **55**:2630–2634.

18. Sweetman SC (Ed) Martindale: The Extra Pharmacopoeia 33rd Edition Pharmaceutical Press London 2002.

19. Hugel H, Ellershaw J, Dickman A. Clonazepam as an adjuvant analgesic in patients with cancer related neuropathic pain. *J Pain Symptom Manage* 2003; **26**:1073–1074.

20. Glynn C. An approach to the management of the patient with deafferentation pain. *Palliat Med* 1989; **3**:13–21.

21. Bartusch SL, Sanders BJ, D'Alessio JG, Jernigan JR. Clonazepam for the treatment of lancinating phantom limb pain. *Clin J Pain* 1996; **12**:59–62.

22. Reddy S, Patt RB. The benzodiazepines as adjuvant analgesics. *J Pain Symptom Manage* 1994; **9**:510–514.

23. Burke AL. Palliative Care: an update on terminal restlessness. *Medical Journal of Australia* 1997; **166**:39–42.

24. Nation RL, Hackett LP, Dusci LJ. Uptake of clonazepam by plastic intravenous infusion bags and administration sets. *Am J Hosp Pharm* 1983; **40**:1692–1693.

25. Hooymans PM, Janknegt R, Lohman JJ. Comparison of clonazepam sorption to polyvinyl chloride-coated and polyethylene-coated tubings. *Pharm Weekbl* 1990; **12**:188–189.

26. Schneider J. Newcastle, Australia. Personal communication (paper in preparation); 2004.

27. Drummond SH, Peterson GM, Galloway JG, Keefe PA. National survey of drug use in palliative care. *Palliat Med* 1996; **10**:119–124.

28. Grassby PF, Hutchings L. Drug combinations in syringe drivers: the compatibility and stability of diamorphine with cyclizine and haloperidol. *Palliat Med* 1997; **11**:217–224.

29. Regnard C, Pashley S, Westrope F. Anti-emetic/diamorphine mixture compatibility in infusion pumps. *Br J Pharm Pract* 1986; **8**:218–220.

30. Walker SE, De Angelis C, Iazzetta J, Eppel JG. Compatibility of dexamethasone sodium phosphate with hydromorphone hydrochloride or diphenhydramine hydrochloride. *Am J Hosp Pharm* 1991; **48**:2161–2166.

31. Hagan RL, Mallett, MS, Fox JL. Stability of ondansetron hydrochloride and dexamethasone sodium phosphate in infusion bags and syringes for 32 days. *Am J Health Syst Pharm* 1996; **53**:1431–1435.

32. Good P, Schneider J, Ravenscroft P. The compatibility and stability of midazolam and dexamethasone in infusion solutions. *J Pain Symptom Manage* 2004; **27**:471–475.

33. Ingallinera TS, Kapadia AJ, Hagman D, Klioze O. Compatibility of glycopyrrolate injection with commonly used infusion solutions and additives. *Am J Hosp Pharm* 1979; **36**:508–510.

34. Page J, Hudson SA. Diamorphine hydrochloride compatibility with saline. *Pharm J* 1982; **228**:238–239.

35. Hain WR, Kirk B. Stability of diamorphine-sodium chloride solutions. *Anaesthesia* 1985; **40**:1241.

36. Beaumont IM. Stability study of aqueous solutions of diamorphine and morphine using HPLC. *Pharm J* 1982; **229**:39–41.

37. Hanks GW, Hoskin PJ, Walker VA. Diamorphine stability and pharmacodynamics. *Anaesthesia* 1987; **42**:664–665.

38. Peterson GM, Randall CT, Paterson J. Plasma levels of morphine and morphine glucuronides in the treatment of cancer pain: relationship to renal function and route of administration. *Eur J Clin Pharmacol* 1990; **38**:121–124.

39. Mercadante S. The role of morphine glucuronides in cancer pain. *Palliat Med* 1999; **13**:95–104.

40. Allwood MC, Brown PW, Lee M. Stability of injections containing diamorphine and midazolam in plastic syringes. *Int J Pharm Pract* 1994; **3**:57–59.

41. Fielding H, Kyaterekera N, Skellern GG, Tettey JN *et al*. The compatibility of octreotide acetate in the presence of diamorphine hydrochloride in polypropylene syringes. *Palliat Med* 2000; **14**(3):205–207.

42. Data on file. GlaxoSmithKline UK Ltd. 2001.

43. Hughes A, Wilcock A, Corcoran R. Ketorolac: Continuous subcutaneous infusion for cancer pain. *J Pain Symptom Manage* 1997; **13**(6):315.

44. Myers KG, Trotman IF. Use of ketorolac by continuous subcutaneous infusion for the control of cancer-related pain. *Postgrad Med J*. 1994; **70**(823):359–62.

45. Dickman A, Ellershaw JE. NSAIDs: gastroprotection or selective COX-2 inhibitor? *Palliat Med* 2004; **18**:275–286.

46. Dollery CT (Ed). Therapeutic Drugs. 2nd Edition Churchill Livingstone, Edinburgh. 1998.

47. Woodruff R. Cancer Pain. Asperula Pty Ltd. Victoria Australia 1997.

48. Bradley K. Swap data on drug compatibilities. *Pharmacy in Pract* 1996; **6**:69–72.

49. Walker SE, Iazzetta J, De Angelis C, Lau DCW. Stability and compatibility of combinations of hydromorphone and dimenhydrinate, lorazepam or prochlorperazine. *Can J Hosp Pharm* 1993; **46**:61–65.

50. Forman JK, Souney PF. Visual compatibility of midazolam hydrochloride with common preoperative injectable medications. *Am J Hosp Pharm* 1987; **44**:2298–2299.

51. Parker WA. Physical compatibilities of preanaesthetic medications. *Can J Hosp Pharm* 1976; **29**:91–92.

52. Dr Paul McIntyre, Halifax, Canada. Personal communication. 2001.

53. Mercadante S, Caligara M, Sapio M, Serretta R *et al*. Subcutaneous fentanyl infusion in a patient with bowel obstruction and renal failure. *J Pain Symptom Manage* 1997; **13**:241–244.

54. Lenz KL, Dunlap DS. Continuous fentanyl infusion: use in severe cancer pain. *Ann Pharmacother* 1998; **32**:316–319.

55. Clotz MA, Nahata MC. Clinical uses of fentanyl, sufentanil and alfentanil. *Clin Pharm* 1991; **10**:581–593.

56. Chandler SW, Trissel LA, Weinstein SM. Combined administration of opioids with selected drugs to manage pain and other cancer symptoms: initial safety screening for compatibility. *J Pain Symptom Manage* 1996; **12**:168–171.

57. Wilson KM, Schneider JJ, Ravenscroft PJ. Stability of midazolam and fentanyl infusion solutions. *J Pain Symptom Manage* 1998; **16**:52–58.

58. Bennett M, Lucas V, Brennan M, Hughes A, O'Donnel V, Wee B. Using anti-muscarinic drugs in the management of death rattle: evidence-based guidelines for palliative care. *Palliat Med* 2002; **16**:369-374.

59. Hugel H. Liverpool UK. Personal communication (paper in preparation). 2004.

60. Davis MP, Furste A. Glycopyrrolate: A Useful Drug in the Palliation of Mechanical Bowel Obstruction. *J Pain Symptom Manage* 1999; **18**:153–154.

61. Huang E, Anderson RP. Compatibility of hydromorphone hydrochloride with haloperidol lactate and ketorolac tromethamine. *Am J Hosp Pharm.* 1994; **51**:2963.

62. Fawcett JP, Woods DJ, Munasiri B, Becket G. Compatibility of cyclizine lactate and haloperidol lactate. *Am J Hosp Pharm* 1994; **51**:2292.

63. Schrijvers D, Tai–Apin C, De Smet MC, Cornil P, Vermorken JB, Bruyneel P. Determination of compatibility and stability of drugs used in palliative care. *J Clin Pharm Ther* 1998; **23**:311–314.

64. Barcia E, Reyes R, Luz Azuara M, Sanchez Y, Negro S. Compatibility of haloperidol and hyoscine-N-butylbromide in mixtures for subcutaneous infusion to cancer patients in palliative care. *Support Care Cancer* 2003; **11**:107–113.

65. De Stoutz ND, Bruera E, Suarez-Almozor M. Opioid rotation for toxicity reduction in terminal cancer patients. *J Pain Symptom Manage* 1995; **10**:378–384.

66. Babul N, Darke AC. Putative role of hydromorphone metabolites in myoclonus. *Pain* 1992; **51**:260–261.

67. Babul N, Darke AC, Hagen N. Hydromorphone metabolite accumulation in renal failure. *J Pain Symptom Manage* 1995; **10**:184–186.

68. Smith MT. Neuroexcitatory effects of morphine and hydromorphone: evidence implicating the 3-glucuronide metabolites. *Clin Exp Pharmacol Physiol* 2000; **27**:524–528.

69. Lee MA, Leng MEF, Tiernan EJJ. Retrospective study of the use of hydromorphone in palliative care patients with normal and abnormal urea and creatinine. *Palliat Med* 2001; **15**:26–34.

70. Lawler P, Turner K, Hanson J, Bruera E. Dose ratio between morphine and hydromorphone in patients with cancer: a retrospective study. *Pain* 1997; **72**:79–85.

71. Bruera E, Pereira J, Watanabe S, Belzile M *et al*. Opioid rotation in patients with cancer pain. A retrospective comparison of dose ratios between methadone, hydromorphone and morphine. *Cancer* 1996; **78**(4):852–857.

72. Storey P, Hill HH, St Louis RH, Tarver EE. Subcutaneous infusions for the control of cancer symptoms. *J Pain Symptom Manage* 1990; **5**(1):33–41.

73. Miller MG, McCarthy N, O'Boyle CA, Kearney M. Continuous subcutaneous infusion of morphine vs. hydromorphone: a controlled trial. *J Pain Symptom Manage* 1999; **18**(1):9–16.

74. Walker SE, Lau DWC. Compatibility and stability of hyaluronidase and hydromorphone. *Can J Hosp Pharm* 1992; **45**:187–192.

75. Trissel LA, Xu Q, Martinez JF, Fox JL. Compatibility and stability of ondansetron hydrochloride with morphine sulphate and with hydromorphone hydrochloride in 0.9% sodium chloride injection at 4, 22 and 32 degrees C. *Am J Hosp Pharm* 1994; **51**(17):2138–2142.

76. Ripamonti C. Management of Bowel Obstruction in Advanced Cancer Patients. *J Pain Symptom Manage* 1994; **9**:193–200.

77. Ripamonti C, Mercadante S, Groff L, Zecca E *et al*. Role of octreotide, scopolamine butylbromide and hydration in symptom control of patients with inoperable bowel obstruction and nasogastric tubes: a prospective randomized trial. *J Pain Symptom Manage* 2000; **19**:23–34.

78. Mercadante S. Scopolamine butylbromide plus octreotide in unresponsive bowel obstruction. *J Pain Symptom Manage* 1998; **16**:278–279.

79. Fallon MT Welsh J. The role of ketamine in pain control. *Eur J Palliat Care* 1996; **3**(4):143–146.

80. Mercadante S, Lodi F, Sapio M, Calligara M *et al*. Long Term Ketamine Subcutaneous Infusion in Neuropathic Cancer Pain. *J Pain Symptom Manage* 1995; **10**:564–568.

81. Wood T, Sloan R. Successful Use of Ketamine for Central Pain. *Palliat Med* 1997; **11**:57–58.

82. Fine PG. Low dose ketamine for the management of opioid non-responsive terminal cancer pain. *J Pain Symptom Manage*. 1999; **17**:296–300.

83. Lloyd –Williams M. Ketamine for cancer pain. *J Pain Symptom Manage* 2000; **19**:79–80.

84. Jackson K, Ashby M, Martin P, Pisasale M, Brumley D, Hayes B. "Burst" ketamine for refractory cancer pain: an open-label audit of 39 patients. *J Pain Symptom Manage* 2001; **22**(4):834–842.

85. Bell RF, Eccleston C, Kalso E. Ketamine as adjuvant to opioids for cancer pain. A qualitative systematic review. *J Pain Symptom Manage* 2003; **26**(3):867–875.

86. Lechner MD, Kreuscher H. [Chemical compatibility of ketamine and midazolam in infusion solutions.] *Anaesthetist* 1990; **39**(1):62–65.

87. Lau MH, Hackman C, Morgan DJ. Compatibility of ketamine and morphine injections. *Pain* 1998; **75**:389–390.

88. Blackwell N, Bangham L, Hughes M, *et al.* Subcutaneous ketorolac - a new development in pain control. *Palliat Med* 1993; **7**:63–65.

89. De Conno F, Zecca E, Martini C, Ripamonti C *et al.* Tolerability of ketorolac administered via continuous subcutaneous infusion for cancer pain: a preliminary report. *J Pain Symptom Manage* 1994; **9**:119–121.

90. Gillis JC, Brogden RN. Ketorolac. A reappraisal of its pharmacodynamic and pharmacokinetic properties and therapeutic use in pain management. *Drugs* 1997; **53**(1):139–188.

91. Twycross RG, Barkby GD, Hallwood PM. The use of low dose methotrimeprazine (levomepromazine) in the management of nausea and vomiting. *Prog Palliat Care* 1997; **5**(2):49–53.

92. Davies A, Mitchell M. Methotrimeprazine and UV light. *Palliat Med* 1996; **10**:264.

93. Gannon C. The use of methadone in the care of the dying. *Eur J Palliat Care* 1997; **4**:152–158.

94. Fitzgibbon DR, Ready LB. Intravenous high-dose methadone administered by patient controlled analgesia and continuous infusion for the treatment of cancer pain refractory to high-dose morphine. *Pain* 1997; **73**:259–261.

95. Mathew P, Storey P. Subcutaneous methadone in terminally ill patients: manageable local toxicity. *J Pain Symptom Manage* 1999; **18**(1):49–52.

96. Makin M, Morley JS. Subcutaneous methadone in terminally ill patients (letter). *J Pain Symptom Manage* 2000; **19**(4):237–238.

97. Thompson DF, Landry JP. Drug-Induced Hiccups. *Ann Pharmacother* 1997; **31**:367–369.

98. Forman JK, Souney PF. Visual compatibility of midazolam hydrochloride with common preoperative injectable medications. *Am J Hosp Pharm* 1987; **44**:2298–2299.

99. Bottomley DM, Hanks GW. Subcutaneous midazolam in palliative care. *J Pain Symptom Manage* 1990; **5**:259–261.

100. Smith GD, Smith MT. Morphine-3-glucuronide: evidence to support its putative role in the development of tolerance to the antinociceptive effects of morphine in rat. *Pain* 1995: **52**:51–60.

101. Hanks GW, De Conno F, Ripamonti C, Ventafridda V *et al.* Morphine in cancer pain: modes of administration. *Br Med J* 1996; **312**:823–826.

102. Hanks GW, Hoskin PJ, Aherne GW, Turner P *et al.* Explanation for potency of repeated oral doses of morphine? *Lancet* 1987; **2**:723–725.

103. Nelson KA, Glare PJ, Walsh D, Groh ES. A prospective, within patient, crossover study of continuous intravenous and subcutaneous morphine for chronic cancer pain. *J Pain Symptom Manage* 1997; **13**:262–267.

104. Lichter I, Hunt E. Drug combinations in syringe drivers. *N Z Med J* 1995; **108**:224–226.

105. Vermeire A, Remon JP, Schrijvers D, Demeulenaere P. A new method to obtain and present complete information on the compatibility: study of its validity for eight binary mixtures of morphine with drugs frequently used in palliative care. *Palliat Med* 2002; **16**:417–424.

106. Mercadante S, Spoldi E, Caraceni A, Maddaloni S *et al.* Octreotide in relieving gastrointestinal symptoms due to bowel obstruction. *Palliat Med* 1993; **7**:295–299.

107. Mangili G, Franchi M, Mariani M, Zanaboni F *et al.* Octreotide in the management of bowel obstruction in terminal ovarian cancer. *Gynecol Oncol* 1996; **61**(3):345–348.

108. Mercadante S, Kargor J, Nicolosi G. Octreotide may prevent definite intestinal obstruction. *J Pain Symptom Manage* 1997; **13**(6): 352–355.

109. Mystakidou K, Tsilika E, Kalaidopoulou O, Chondros K, Georgaki S, Papadimitriou L. Comparison of octreotide administration vs conservative treatment in the management of inoperable bowel obstruction in patients with far advanced cancer: a randomized, double- blind, controlled clinical trial. *Anticancer Res* 2002; **22**(2B):1187–1192.

110. Mercadante S, Ripamonti C, Casuccio A, Zecca E, Groff L. Comparison of octreotide and hyoscine butylbromide in controlling gastrointestinal symptoms due to malignant inoperable bowel obstruction. *Support Care Cancer* 2000; **8**(3):188–191.

111. Riley J, Fallon MT. Octreotide in terminal malignant obstruction of the gastrointestinal tract. *Eur J Palliat Care* 1994; **1**(1):23–25.

112. Mulvenna PM, Regnard CFB. Subcutaneous Ondansetron. *Lancet* 1992; **339**:1059.

113. Currow DC, Coughlan M, Fardell B, *et al.* Use of Ondansetron in Palliative Medicine. *J Pain Symptom Manage* 1997; **13**(5):302–307.

114. Kyriakides K, Hussain SK, Hobbs GJ. Management of opioid-induced pruritus: a role for 5-HT3 antagonists? *Br J Anaesth* 1999; **82**:439–441.

115. Lonsdale-Eccles A, Carmichael AJ. Treatment of pruritus associated with systemic disorders in the elderly: a review of the role of new therapies. *Drugs Aging* 2003; **20**:197–208.

116. Murphy M, Reaich D, Pai P, Finn P, Carmichael AJ. A randomized, placebo-controlled, double-blind trial of ondansetron in renal itch. *Br J Dermatol* 2003; **148**:314–317.

117. Muller C, Pongratz S, Pidlich J, Penner E *et al.* Treatment of pruritus in chronic liver disease with the 5-hydroxytryptamine receptor type 3

antagonist ondansetron: a randomized, placebo-controlled, double-blind cross-over trial. *Eur J Gastroenterol Hepatol* 1998; **10**:865–870.

118. Arcioni R, della Rocca M, Romano S, Romano R, Pietropaoli P, Gasparetto A. Ondansetron inhibits the analgesic effects of tramadol: a possible 5-HT(3) spinal receptor involvement in acute pain in humans. *Anesth Analg* 2002; **94**:1553–1557.

119. Ross FB, Smith MT. The intrinsic antinociceptive effects of oxycodone appear to be kappa-opioid receptor mediated. *Pain* 1997; **73**:151–157.

120. Heiskanen T, Olkkola KT, Kalso E. Effects of blocking CYP2D6 on the pharmacokinetics and pharmacodynamics of oxycodone. *Clin Pharmacol Ther* 1998; **64**:603–611.

121. Smith MT, Ross FB, Nielsen CK, Saini K. Oxycodone has a distinctly different pharmacology from morphine. *Eur J Pain* 2001; **5**(S1): 135–136.

122. Kaiko RF, Benziger DP, Fitzmartin RD, Burke BE, Reder RF, Goldenheim PD. Clinical pharmacokinetics of controlled released oxycodone in renal impairment. *Clin Pharmacol Ther.* 1996; **59**:52–61.

123. Kirvela M, Lindgren L, Seppala T, Olkkola KT. The pharmacokinetics of oxycodone in uremic patients undergoing renal transplantation. *J Clin Anesth.* 1996; **8**:13–18.

124. Gardiner PR. Compatibility of an oxycodone injectable formulation with typical diluents, syringes, tubings, infusion bags and drugs for potential co-administration. *Hospital Pharmacist* 2003; **10**:354–361.

125. Dickman A, Hunter S. Compatibility of oxycodone with palliative care supportive drugs. (Paper in preparation) 2004.

126. Stirling LC, Kurowska A, Tookman A. The use of phenobarbitone in the management of agitation and seizures at the end of life. *J Pain Symptom Manage* 1999; **17**:363–8.

127. Knapp AJ, Mauro VF, Alexander KS. Incompatibility of ketorolac tromethamine with selective postoperative drugs. *Am J Hosp Pharm* 1992; **49**:2960–2962.

128. Dr Frank Formby, Wollongong, Australia. Personal communication. 2004.

129. Reymond L, Charles MA, Bowman J, Treston P. The effect of dexamethasone on the longevity of syringe driver subcutaneous sites in palliative care patients. *MJA* 2003; **178**:486–489.

130. Parker WA. Physical compatibility of ranitidine HCl with preoperative injectable medications. *Can J Hosp Pharm* 1985; **38**:160–161.

131. Raffa RB, Friderichs E, Reimann W, Shank RP, Codd EE, Vaught JL. Opioid and nonopioid components independently contribute to the mechanism of action if tramadol, an 'atypical' opioid analgesic. *J Pharmacol Exp Ther* 1992; **260**:275–285.

132. Raffa RB, Friderichs E, Reimann W, Shank RP et al. Complementary and synergistic antinociceptive interaction between the enantiomers of tramadol. *J Pharmacol Exp Ther* 1993; **267**:331–340.

133. Desmeules JA, Piguet V, Collart L, Dayer P. Contribution of monoaminergic modulation to the analgesic effect of tramadol. *Br J Clin Pharmacol.* 1996; **41**:7–12.

134. Collart L, Luthy C, Favario-Constantin C, Dayer P. Duality of analgesic effect of tramadol in man. *Schweiz-Med-Wochenschr* 1993; **123**:2241–2243.

135. Duhmke R, Cornblath D, Hollingshead J. Tramadol for neuropathic pain. *Cochrane Database Syst Rev.* 2004; **2**:CD003726.

136. Webb AR, Leong S, Myles PS, Burn SJ. The addition of a tramadol infusion to morphine patient-controlled analgesia after abdominal surgery: a double-blinded, placebo-controlled randomized trial. *Anesth Analg* 2002; **95**:1713–1718.

Chapter 3

Symptom control with the syringe driver

Introduction

Palliative care patients often exhibit multiple pathologies which generally require the use of numerous drug treatments. As the patient's condition deteriorates, the oral route may no longer be feasible, hence an alternative method is required. A CSCI, via the syringe driver, provides a simple and effective way to control symptoms. This chapter discusses how CSCIs can be used in the treatment of several distressing symptoms. Refer to the monographs in Chapter 2 for additional drug information.

Important note The maximum volume of a PRN subcutaneous injection is 2 ml; above this value, the injection will be painful for the patient and therefore a further site must be used.

Pain

The dose of opioid to infuse depends upon previous requirements. Refer to Tables 2.2, 2.3 and 2.4 for equianalgesic ratios and conversion tables. Unresolved nociceptive and neuropathic pains may give rise to terminal agitation and must be anticipated; patients may also have an exacerbation of pain at this time. Figures 3.1 and 3.2 provide simple algorithms of the points discussed below.

If the patient was previously taking a modified release (m/r) oral opioid, the driver should be started at the time the next dose is due. For practical purposes, a crossover period is generally not considered necessary. However, some practitioners recommend starting the driver four hours prior to the next m/r dose. In either case, to achieve or maintain adequate analgesia, a suitable subcutaneous bolus dosage may be required.

If the patient is currently using a transdermal buprenorphine or fentanyl patch, treatment should continue with this formulation. Breakthrough pain should be treated with equivalent 'rescue' doses of subcutaneous opioid (refer to Table 2.3). The total daily rescue medication is then given via a CSCI, in addition to the transdermal patch. A study concluded that continuation with the fentanyl patch in this manner did not compromise analgesia;[1] there is no reason to assume that this would not happen with the buprenorphine patch.

If the patient receives rescue medication for incident pain (i.e. agitation or pain on movement), this is not an indication to increase the daily dose of analgesia. Since the patient experiencing incident pain is not suffering while at rest, any rescue dose of opioid given must *not* be included when calculating the new daily analgesia dose. This simple measure should prevent the rapid development of opioid toxicity. It would be sensible to prescribe a separate opioid treatment, if possible, on the prescription for incident pain, to avoid this confusion.

A suitable starting point for the treatment of incident pain is the administration of a SC rescue dose of opioid, coupled with 2.5 to 5 mg SC *midazolam* at least 15 minutes prior to movement. Midazolam is used to induce a state of amnesia, a useful effect of midazolam, employed in surgery. However, rescue doses of diamorphine, morphine, hydromorphone or oxycodone will produce an effect that will persist for several hours, even after the incident pain has subsided; this excess of opioid could manifest in the form of drowsiness, confusion, or possibly agitation. *Alfentanil*, at a suitable equianalgesic dose, can be administered for incident pain, particularly as it has such a short duration of action.

Neuropathic pain is believed to be only partially responsive to opioid analgesia; hence, the concurrent use of adjuvant analgesics. Unfortunately, most adjuvants cannot be given via CSCI. *Clonazepam* can be considered, whilst some specialists may contemplate the use of *ketamine* or *methadone*. Clonazepam should be considered (at an initial dose of 2–4 mg) if the patient is being treated for neuropathic pain, preferably before symptoms of pain become apparent. Note that clonazepam can also be effective in the control of terminal agitation; as such, the concurrent use of midazolam is not recommended in this situation.

Important note Loss of clonazepam using PVC giving sets has been reported. The clinical significance is unknown, but given the high adsorption rate, the first infusion through new tubing may not produce the anticipated response. This fact must be borne in mind when assessing the treatment and before increasing the dose. It is advisable to use non-PVC tubing, if clonazepam has to be infused.

Ketamine and methadone should only be initiated at specialist centres; in the latter case, the patient should be stabilized on oral methadone before attempting conversion to a CSCI. For nerve compression pain, dexamethasone 8–16 mg may be considered for 48–72 hours. Note that dexamethasone is usually administered in one or two divided doses, rather than via a CSCI.

Renal failure can precipitate diamorphine/morphine toxicity, due to the accumulation of the metabolites, M3G and M6G.[2] Generally, if the patient clearly shows signs of opioid toxicity, the dose should be reduced by 30%. The rescue dosage must also be amended. If the patient is not pain-controlled after this reduction, opioid rotation should be considered; *alfentanil* is the recommended as an alternative (*sufentanil* can be considered, where available). Oxycodone also accumulates in renal failure; however oxycodone does not have such problematic metabolites, so careful reduction of the dose should prevent the need for opioid rotation. Fentanyl cannot readily be considered for use via the syringe driver because of its volume constraints. A renally excreted metabolite of *hydromorphone* may accumulate and may cause similar problems as morphine; a dosage reduction may prevent the need for opioid rotation.

Bone pain is also difficult to treat with opioids alone. Generally, this can be successfully controlled with the use of an NSAID via a CSCI. *Ketorolac* is the recommended drug, although *diclofenac* has been used. These will more than likely necessitate the use of a second syringe driver and the dose of any concurrent opioid must be reviewed. The practicalities of using a proton pump inhibitor must be considered. In rare situations where a NSAID is contra-indicated, *tramadol* can be considered, in addition to any concurrent opioid. As with NSAIDs, the dose of a concurrent opioid must be reviewed. *Dexamethasone* can be used to treat bone pain, although this is rare.

Pain associated with bowel obstruction should be treated with an antimuscarinic, such as *glycopyrronium*. If other smooth muscle spasm is suspected (e.g. renal colic, biliary colic) the use of a NSAID such as *ketorolac* or *diclofenac* may be considered.

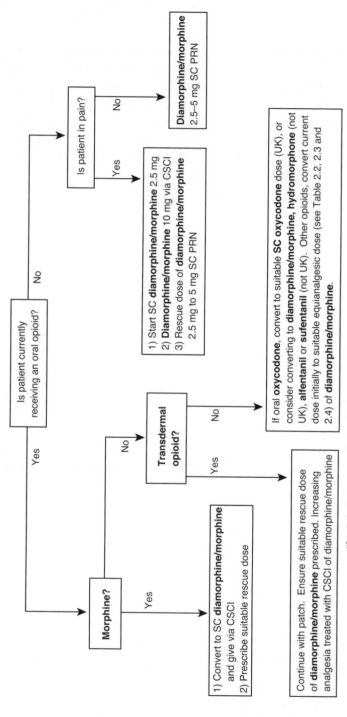

Is patient currently receiving an oral opioid?

Yes → **Morphine?**
No → **Is patient in pain?**

Is patient in pain?
- **Yes** →
  1) Start SC **diamorphine/morphine** 2.5 mg
  2) **Diamorphine/morphine** 10 mg via CSCI
  3) Rescue dose of **diamorphine/morphine** 2.5 mg to 5 mg SC PRN
- **No** → **Diamorphine/morphine** 2.5–5 mg SC PRN

Morphine?
- **Yes** →
  1) Convert to SC **diamorphine/morphine** and give via CSCI
  2) Prescribe suitable rescue dose
- **No** → **Transdermal opioid?**

Transdermal opioid?
- **Yes** → Continue with patch. Ensure suitable rescue dose of **diamorphine/morphine** prescribed. Increasing analgesia treated with CSCI of diamorphine/morphine
- **No** → If oral **oxycodone**, convert to suitable **SC oxycodone** dose (UK), or consider converting to **diamorphine/morphine**, **hydromorphone** (not UK), **alfentanil** or **sufentanil** (not UK). Other opioids, convert current dose initially to suitable equianalgesic dose (see Table 2.2, 2.3 and 2.4) of **diamorphine/morphine**.

Fig. 3.1 Recommended opioid treatment for a patient requiring a syringe driver.

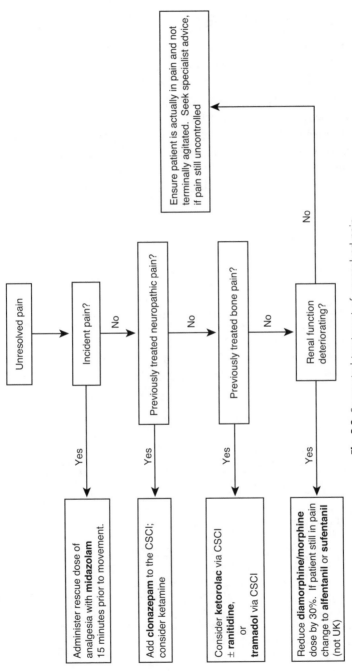

Fig. 3.2 Suggested treatment of unresolved pain.

Nausea and Vomiting

One of the indications for a CSCI is uncontrolled nausea and vomiting. Nausea usually precedes vomiting and can be described as 'the unpleasant sensation associated with the urge to vomit'. Gastric stasis generally accompanies nausea, so an initial parenteral dose of an antiemetic should be considered.

The main neuropharmacological pathways involved in the emetic process should be understood, in order to ensure optimal pharmacological intervention (see Fig. 3.3). There is an area of the brain located in the reticular formation of the lower medulla that appears to control

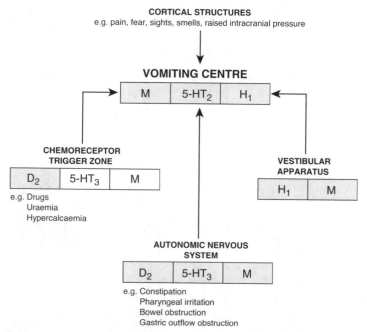

Fig. 3.3 Causes of nausea and vomiting. The shaded boxes represent prominent pharmacological targets.

the complex act of vomiting; this is the vomiting centre. Emesis occurs when the vomiting centre receives impulses from the following:

♦ Chemoreceptor trigger zone (CTZ)

♦ Vestibular apparatus

♦ Higher centres of the brain (cerebral cortex and limbic system)

♦ Autonomic nervous system (for example, pharynx, gastrointestinal tract, visceral organs)

The CTZ is located in the area postrema in the floor of the fourth ventricle and lies outside the blood–brain diffusion barrier. It is stimulated by emetogenic substances borne by both blood and cerebrospinal fluid. The principal emetogenic pathway appears to involve dopamine type 2 (D_2) receptors, although serotonin type 3 (5-HT_3) and acetylcholine muscarinic (M) receptors are also involved. The nucleus tractus solitarius is the main site for peripheral input from autonomic afferent neurones. D_2, 5-HT_3 and M receptors are potential targets here. Impulses from the vestibular apparatus pass through the vestibular nucleus where histamine type 1 (H_1) and M receptors represent the pharmacological targets. Receptors within the vomiting centre include serotonin type 2 (5-HT_2), H_1 and M. Incidentally, μ-receptors are located in the CTZ (potentially emetic) and vomiting centre (potentially antiemetic).[3] This would suggest that lipophilic opioids, such as alfentanil and fentanyl, may theoretically cause less nausea and vomiting than hydrophilic opioids such as morphine.

A thorough assessment and history is vital in order to identify the cause(s) of nausea and vomiting, as well as to enable the most suitable choice of antiemetic. Some of the common causes of nausea and vomiting encountered in palliative care are shown in Box 3.1.

Box 3.1 Possible causes of nausea and vomiting

♦ Drugs (e.g. opioids, cytotoxics, antibiotics, digoxin, iron, NSAIDs)	♦ Stress/anxiety	♦ Constipation
	♦ Gastric ulceration	♦ Renal failure
	♦ Bowel obstruction	♦ Hypercalcaemia
♦ Gastroparesis	♦ Bowel colic	♦ Raised intracranial pressure

Antiemetics

The choice of an antiemetic will depend on the cause(s) of nausea and vomiting. Most patients, however, have multiple and often irreversible causes. Figure 3.4 illustrates the areas of the vomiting pathway where certain drugs act. Antiemetics may act at more than one type of receptor in producing their effect. For example, cyclizine may interact at both M and H_1 receptors; levomepromazine acts at 5-HT_2, D_2, H_1, M receptors. Currently, no available drug will antagonize all receptor sites involved in the vomiting pathway, nor is there a universal agent that will block the final common pathway, the output from the vomiting centre. Consequently, a combination of agents may

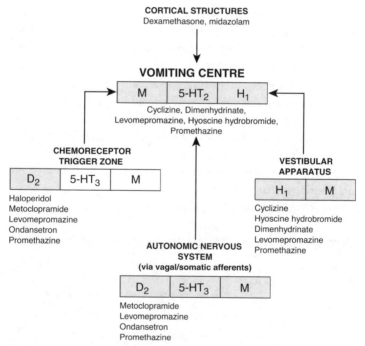

Fig. 3.4 Sites of action of selected antiemetics. The shaded boxes represent prominent pharmacological targets.

have a greater antiemetic action than a single drug. The drugs chosen should have synergistic, rather than additive or opposing pharmacological actions. For example, ondansetron and levomepromazine is a suitable combination because all the recognized receptors involved in the process are covered; haloperidol and metoclopramide is not a sensible combination because of the increased risk of extrapyramidal reactions. For resistant cases of nausea and vomiting, Table 3.1 should facilitate the choice of a suitable antiemetic. However, in general:

- *Levomepromazine* 6.25–12.5 mg by SC injection at night should be considered in resistant cases.[4]

- In case large volumes are being vomited, a combination of anti-secretory drugs such as *octreotide* 500 micrograms and *glycopyrronium* 1.2 mg or *hyoscine butylbromide* 120 mg can be considered.[5,6]

- *Ondansetron* is a suitable second or third line choice; it may be beneficial only if the cause of nausea/vomiting is due to renal failure or damage to gastrointestinal enterochromaffin cells, i.e. recent radiotherapy/chemotherapy, bowel obstruction, gastric cancers.

- *Dexamethasone* can be used in difficult cases and often produces an indirect antiemetic effect, particularly in bowel obstruction, by reducing inflammatory oedema around the tumour or improving peristalsis. It may also have an 'as-yet-unproven direct antiemetic effect'.

Restlessness and agitation

General points

Terminal restlessness can be described as 'agitated delirium in a dying patient, frequently associated with impaired consciousness and myoclonic events.' Patients can suffer symptoms of agitation, moaning/crying out, physical restlessness, myoclonic spasms, or convulsions. Its presence can be distressing for both family and carer and may leave unpleasant, negative memories of an otherwise, fairly peaceful dying process. The cause of terminal restlessness could be

Table 3.1 Suggested treatments of nausea and vomiting using either a CSCI or subcutaneous injections

Cause	First-line drug	Stat dose	Daily dose	Second-line drug[1]	Stat dose	Daily dose	Notes
Gastric stasis	**Metoclopramide**	10 mg	30–120 mg	–	–	–	Antimuscarinic drugs and 5-HT$_3$ antagonists may reduce the prokinetic effect
Gastric irritation (e.g. drugs, tumour infiltration)	**Metoclopramide**	10 mg	30–120 mg	**Levomepromazine** or **Ondansetron**[2]	6.25 mg 8 mg	6.25–25 mg 24–32 mg	Consider oral proton pump inhibitor, if possible, or a CSCI of **ranitidine** 150–300 mg if NSAID induced.
Total bowel obstruction with colic	**Haloperidol** or **Promethazine**[3] and consider **Hyoscine butylbromide** or **Glycopyrronium**	1.5–5 mg 25–50 mg 20 mg 400 micrograms	5–10 mg 50–150 mg 80–160 mg 800–2400 micrograms	**Add cyclizine** or **Dimenhydrinate**[4] **Levomepromazine** **Ondansetron**[2]	50 mg 25–50 mg 6.25 mg 8 mg	100–150 mg 50–200 mg 6.25–25 mg (CSCI or SC stat) 24–32 mg	In difficult cases, consider the use of **dexamethasone** 8–12 mg daily (SC) and review after 5 days. **Octreotide** 300–600 µg daily (CSCI) with **glycopyrronium** may be beneficial if large volume vomit.
Partial bowel obstruction without colic	**Metoclopramide**	10 mg	30–120 mg	**Add dexamethasone**	8–12 mg	8–12 mg (CSCI or SC stat)	Consider faecal softner (e.g. **docusate sodium** 100 mg bd)

Cause	First line			Second line			Comments
Chemoreceptor trigger zone (e.g. drugs, hypercalcaemia)	Haloperidol	1.5–5 mg	5–10 mg	Add cyclizine	50 mg	150 mg	
	or Metoclopramide	50 mg	150 mg	or Add dimenhydrinate[4]	25–50 mg	50–200 mg	
	or Promethazine[3]	25–50 mg	50–150 mg	or Levomepromazine	6.25 mg	6.25–25 mg (CSCI or SC stat)	
Raised intracranial pressure	Dexamethasone and either	8–16 mg	8–16 mg (CSCI or SC stat)	Levomepromazine and dexamethasone	6.25 mg	6.25–25 mg (CSCI or SC stat)	Do not administer dexamethasone and levomepromazine together via the same CSCI.
	Cyclizine	50 mg	150 mg				
	or Dimenhydrinate[4]	25–50 mg	50–200 mg				
	or Promethazine	25–50 mg	50–150 mg				

[1] Substitute the first line drug with the second line agent *unless* the table states otherwise.

[2] Useful if problem due to cellular damage with subsequent serotonin release e.g. radiotherapy, renal failure.

[3] Not generally considered in UK. Is used successfully in Australia, where cyclizine is not readily obtainable. Ensure promethazine is not co-prescribed with other D_2, or H_1 receptor antagonists.

[4] Not available in the UK. Is a suitable alternative to cyclizine in Canada and USA.

Box 3.2 Suggested causes of terminal agitation

♦ drugs (note that previously tolerated doses of drugs, especially morphine, may become toxic as the patient's renal/liver function deteriorates.)

♦ pain,

♦ brain tumour/metastases,

♦ hypercalcaemia/hyponatraemia/hypoglycaemia,

♦ renal failure/liver failure,

♦ constipation,

♦ urinary retention,

♦ infection,

♦ nicotine/alcohol withdrawal and

♦ emotional distress (e.g. fear, anxiety).

multifactorial; several causes are shown in Box 3.2. For patients close to death, it is generally inappropriate to investigate and treat the metabolic or infective causes. However, other causes that can be considered to be 'reversible' (underlined in Box 3.2) should be managed accordingly.

Management

A suggested management plan has been described here and outlined in Fig. 3.5.

1 Check to see if a 'reversible' cause, as outlined above, can be identified and treat accordingly.

e.g. if the patient has suddenly stopped smoking, consider the use of a *nicotine* patch;

if opioid toxicity is suspected due to worsening renal function, consider changing diamorphine/morphine to alfentanil.

2 Ensure that SC PRN doses of *midazolam* (e.g. 2.5 mg–10 mg) are prescribed for breakthrough agitation/anxiety.

3 Begin titrating the dose of midazolam. If two or more PRN doses are administered in a 24-hour period, consider adding to, or commencing a CSCI. Continue to administer appropriate PRN doses and review requirements daily. If oxycodone is currently prescribed via CSCI, *clonazepam* would be a more suitable choice due to volume restrictions. However, midazolam should be continued for PRN doses.

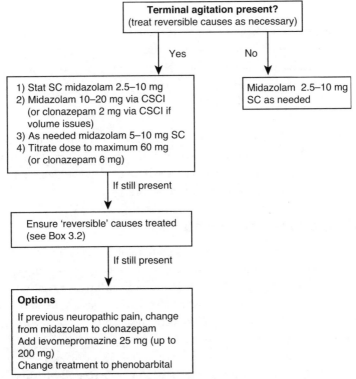

Fig. 3.5 Suggested treatment of terminal agitation.

4 For more resistant forms of terminal restlessness, the following is suggested, in order:

(i) if previous neuropathic pain, change midazolam in the CSCI to *clonazepam* (use 2 mg, if less than 20 mg midazolam in 24 hours). The dose may need to be increased as necessary, up to 6-8 mg. Continue with midazolam for stat doses. Note that the doses quoted above are arbitrary, and do not represent dose equivalences between the benzodiazepines;

(ii) Add *levomepromazine* 25 mg to the driver (check for compatibility). The dosage can be increased as necessary (usually in 25–50 mg increments, depending on severity) up to a maximum of 200 mg. This drug is reserved as a second line agent because of the potential for myoclonus. It is a useful adjunct to a benzodiazepine for uncontrolled agitation.

Important note If midazolam or levomepromazine are unavailable, suitable alternatives include promethazine, hyoscine hydrobromide, haloperidol and phenobarbital. Note however, that the former two drugs can cause paradoxical agitation.

(iii) In the event that the above measures fail to control symptoms, change to phenobarbital 200 mg via CSCI over 24 hours. This must be given via a separate driver. The dose can be increased, if necessary, to 1200 mg.

Respiratory tract secretions

Drugs will not be able to 'dry-up' secretions already present; hence, it is important that the treatment is initiated as soon as symptoms appear. The 'death rattle' is usually more disturbing for relatives or carers than the patient, who is usually semi-conscious. In addition to patient positioning, the pharmacological options via CSCI over 24 hours include *glycopyrronium* 0.6–2.4 mg, *hyoscine hydrobromide* 1.2–2.4 mg and *hyoscine butylbromide* 20–180 mg (see Fig. 3.6). Glycopyrronium is generally preferred due to perceived pharmacological benefits and cost effectiveness. Note, however, that there is

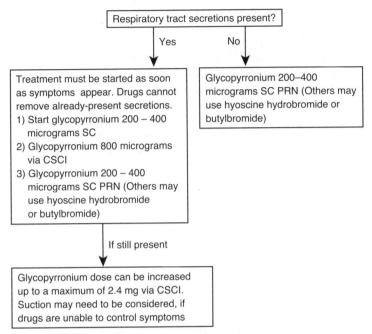

Fig. 3.6 Suggested treatment of terminal secretions.

no evidence to support the superiority of any one drug. Stat doses must be prescribed for breakthrough secretions. Some centres use hyoscine butylbromide as a first line choice because it is cheaper than glycopyrronium, but possibly not as effective.

Volume of glycopyrronium injection is likely to be the main problem encountered with the treatment of this condition. The maximum 2.4 mg dose of glycopyrronium equates to 12 ml of liquid. The Graseby MS26 can infuse a maximum of between 20–22 ml (using a 30 ml syringe). It is possible that the total volume to be infused will exceed this amount. In such cases, a twelve-hourly infusion rate will be needed.

References

1. Ellershaw JE, Kinder C, Aldridge J, Allison M, Smith JC. Care of the dying: is pain control compromised or enhanced by continuation of the fentanyl transdermal patch in the dying phase? *J Pain Symptom Manage*. 2002; **24**:398–403.

2. Mercadante S. The role of morphine glucuronides in cancer pain. *Palliat Med* 1999; **13**:95–104.

3. Twycross RG, Wilcock A. Symptom Management in Advanced Cancer. Third Edition. Radcliffe Medical Press. Oxford. UK 2001.

4. Twycross RG, Barkby GD, Hallwood PM. The use of low dose methotrimeprazine (levomepromazine) in the management of nausea and vomiting. *Progress in Palliative Care* 1997; **5**(2):49–53.

5. Mercadante S. Scopolamine butylbromide plus octreotide in unresponsive bowel obstruction. *J Pain Symptom Manage* 1998; **16**:278–279.

6. Davis MP, Furste A. Glycopyrrolate: A Useful Drug in the Palliation of Mechanical Bowel Obstruction. *J Pain Symptom Manage* 1999; **18**:153–154.

Chapter 4

Compatibility Data Tables

Stability information presented here comes from laboratory work and the clinical setting. Where possible, data from the literature have been included. Please note that compatibility shown here does not imply stability at different concentrations.

In the following tables, the convention as shown in the key below has been adopted. Also note that, unless otherwise stated, diamorphine is reconstituted with 1 ml WFI and clonazepam is not diluted with the supplied WFI.

Key

DEX	Dextrose 5% in water
NaCl	Sodium chloride 0.9%
WFI	Water for Injections
$\checkmark_{(P)}$	Mixture physically compatible for the time shown
$\checkmark_{(PC)}$ (24 hours)	Mixture chemically and physically compatible for the time shown
✗	Mixture incompatible
CLIN	Clinical observation
LAB	Laboratory study

Compatibility data tables

Two Drugs

Drug A	B	Page
Alfentanil	Clonazepam	120
Alfentanil	Cyclizine	120
Alfentanil	Dexamethasone	120
Alfentanil	Glycopyrronium	121
Alfentanil	Haloperidol	121
Alfentanil	Hyoscine Butylbromide	121
Alfentanil	Levomepromazine	121
Alfentanil	Metoclopramide	122
Alfentanil	Midazolam	122
Alfentanil	Ondansetron	122
Diamorphine	Cyclizine	122
Diamorphine	Dexamethasone	124
Diamorphine	Haloperidol	125
Diamorphine	Hyoscine Butylbromide	126
Diamorphine	Hyoscine Hydrobromide	126
Diamorphine	Ketorolac	127
Diamorphine	Levomepromazine	127
Diamorphine	Metoclopramide	128
Diamorphine	Midazolam	129
Diamorphine	Octreotide	130
Diamorphine	Ondansetron	130
Dihydrocodeine	Cyclizine	131
Dihydrocodeine	Dexamethasone	131
Dihydrocodeine	Haloperidol	131
Dihydrocodeine	Levomepromazine	132
Fentanyl	Dexamethasone	132
Fentanyl	Haloperidol	132
Fentanyl	Hyoscine Hydrobromide	132
Fentanyl	Ketamine	133

Drug A	B	Page
Fentanyl	Levomepromazine	133
Fentanyl	Metoclopramide	133
Fentanyl	Midazolam	134
Fentanyl	Ondansetron	134
Hydromorphone	Dimenhydrinate	135
Hydromorphone	Haloperidol	135
Hydromorphone	Midazolam	135
Methadone	Clonazepam	136
Methadone	Midazolam	136
Morphine Hydrochloride	Dexamethasone	136
Morphine Hydrochloride	Haloperidol	137
Morphine Hydrochloride	Hyoscine Butylbromide	137
Morphine Hydrochloride	Metoclopramide	137
Morphine Hydrochloride	Midazolam	137
Morphine Sulphate	Cyclizine	138
Morphine Sulphate	Haloperidol	138
Morphine Sulphate	Metoclopramide	139
Morphine Sulphate	Ondansetron	139
Morphine Tartrate	Dexamethasone	139
Morphine Tartrate	Haloperidol	140
Morphine Tartrate	Metoclopramide	140
Oxycodone	Clonazepam	140
Oxycodone	Cyclizine	141
Oxycodone	Dexamethasone	141
Oxycodone	Haloperidol	142

Drug A	B	Page	Drug A	B	Page
Oxycodone	Hyoscine Butylbromide	142	Dexamethasone	Hyoscine Hydrobromide	150
Oxycodone	Hyoscine Hydrobromide	142	Dexamethasone	Levomepromazine	151
			Dexamethasone	Metoclopramide	151
Oxycodone	Ketamine	143	Dexamethasone	Midazolam	152
Oxycocone	Ketorolac	143			
Oxycodone	Levomepromazine	143	Dexamethasone	Promethazine	152
			Dimenhydrinate	Glycopyrronium	153
Oxycodone	Metoclopramide	144	Glycopyrronium	Ondansetron	153
Oxycodone	Midazolam	144	Glycopyrronium	Ranitidine	153
Oxycodone	Octreotide	144	Haloperidol	Hyoscine Butylbromide	154
Oxycodone	Ondansetron	145			
Oxycodone	Ranitidine	145	Haloperidol	Ketamine	154
Tramadol	Dexamethasone	145	Haloperidol	Metoclopramide	154
Tramadol	Haloperidol	146	Haloperidol	Midazolam	154
Tramadol	Hyoscine Butylbromide	146	Hyoscine Butylbromide	Midazolam	155
Tramadol	Metoclopramide	146			
Tramadol	Midazolam	146	Ketamine	Midazolam	155
Clonazepam	Dexamethasone	147	Ketorolac	Ranitidine	155
Clonazepam	Glycopyrronium	147	Levomepromazine	Octreotide	156
Clonazepam	Haloperidol	147	Levomepromazine	Ranitidine	156
Clonazepam	Metoclopramide	148	Metoclopramide	Midazolam	156
Cyclizine	Dexamethasone	148	Metoclopramide	Octreotide	157
Cyclizine	Haloperidol	148	Metoclopramide	Ondansetron	157
Cyclizine	Metoclopramide	149	Midazolam	Ondansetron	157
Dexamethasone	Haloperidol	149	Octreotide	Ondansetron	157
Dexamethasone	Hyoscine Butylbromide	150			

Alfentanil (A) and Clonazepam (B)

Summary: No problems with physical stability encountered. Loss of clonazepam observed when infused via PVC tubing.[1] Minimize loss by using non-PVC tubing.

Drug	Dose in syringe (mg)	Volume in syringe (ml)	Concentration (mg/ml)	Diluent	Outcome	Data Type
A	80	20	4.00	–	✓(P) (24 h)	LAB
B	4		0.20			

Alfentanil (A) and Cyclizine (B)

Summary: Problems with physical compatibility are likely as concentrations of either drug increase (compare diamorphine/cyclizine).

Drug	Dose in syringe (mg)	Volume in syringe (ml)	Concentration (mg/ml)	Diluent	Outcome	Data Type
A	2	17	0.12	WFI	✓(P) (24 h)	CLIN
B	150		8.82			
A	4	17	0.24	WFI	✓(P) (24 h)	CLIN
B	150		8.82			
A	85	20	4.25	–	✗	LAB
B	150		7.50			

Alfentanil (A) and Dexamethasone (B)

Summary: No problems with physical stability encountered. Dexamethasone is usually given as a subcutaneous bolus injection (depending upon volume of injection) or via a separate CSCI. However, if dexamethasone is to be mixed with other drugs, it should be the last constituent added to the maximally diluted syringe. There may be initial transient turbidity upon the addition of dexamethasone.

Drug	Dose in syringe (mg)	Volume in syringe (ml)	Concentration (mg/ml)	Diluent	Outcome	Data Type
A	80	20	4.00	–	✓(P) (24 h)	LAB
B	16		0.80			

Alfentanil (A) and Glycopyrronium (B)

Summary: No problems with physical stability encountered.

Drug	Dose in syringe (mg)	Volume in syringe (ml)	Concentration (mg/ml)	Diluent	Outcome	Data Type
A	60	20	3.00	–	✓ (P) (24 h)	LAB
B	1.6		0.08			

Alfentanil (A) and Haloperidol (B)

Summary: No problems with physical stability encountered.

Drug	Dose in syringe (mg)	Volume in syringe (ml)	Concentration (mg/ml)	Diluent	Outcome	Data Type
A	85	20	4.25	–	✓ (P) (24 h)	LAB
B	15		0.75			

Alfentanil (A) and Hyoscine Buytlbromide (B)

Summary: No problems with physical stability encountered.

Drug	Dose in syringe (mg)	Volume in syringe (ml)	Concentration (mg/ml)	Diluent	Outcome	Data Type
A	70	20	3.50	–	✓ (P) (24 h)	LAB
B	120		6.00			

Alfentanil (A) and Levomepromazine (B)

Summary: No problems with physical stability encountered. To avoid irritation at the site of infusion, levomepromazine may be given as a subcutaneous bolus injection at doses below 50 mg (= 2ml).

Drug	Dose in syringe (mg)	Volume in syringe (ml)	Concentration (mg/ml)	Diluent	Outcome	Data Type
A	3	8	0.38	WFI	✓ (P) (24 h)	CLIN
B	12.5		1.56			
A	90	20	4.50	–	✓ (P) (24 h)	LAB
B	50		2.50			

Alfentanil (A) and Metoclopramide (B)

Summary: No problems with physical stability encountered.

Drug	Dose in syringe (mg)	Volume in syringe (ml)	Concentration (mg/ml)	Diluent	Outcome Type	Data
A	60	20	3.00	–	✔ (P) (24 h)	LAB
B	40		2.00			

Alfentanil (A) and Midazolam (B)

Summary: No problems with physical stability encountered.

Drug	Dose in syringe (mg)	Volume in syringe (ml)	Concentration (mg/ml)	Diluent	Outcome	Data Type
A	3	10	0.30	WFI	✔ (P) (24 h)	CLIN
B	30		3.00			
A	60	20	3.00	–	✔ (P) (24 h)	LAB
B	40		2.00			

Alfentanil (A) and Ondansetron (B)

Summary: No problems with physical stability encountered.

Drug	Dose in syringe (mg)	Volume in syringe (ml)	Concentration (mg/ml)	Diluent	Outcome	Data Type
A	6	35	0.17	NaCl	✔ (P) (24 h)	LAB[2]
B	46.5		1.33			

Diamorphine (A) and Cyclizine (B)

Summary: Physically and chemically[3,4,5] compatible as shown below, although crystallization can occur as concentrations increase. If the diamorphine concentration exceeds 20 mg/ml, crystallization may occur unless the concentration of cyclizine is *no greater than* 10 mg/ml. Similarly, if the concentration of cyclizine exceeds 20 mg/ml, crystallization may occur unless the concentration of diamorphine is *no greater than* 15 mg/ml.

Drug	Dose in syringe (mg)	Volume in syringe (ml)	Concentration (mg/ml)	Diluent	Outcome	Data Type
A	20	17	1.18	WFI	✓ (P) (24 h)	CLIN
B	150		8.82			
A	40	17	2.35	WFI	✓ (P) (24 h)	CLIN
B	150		8.82			
A	100	17	5.88	WFI	✓ (PC) (24 h)	LAB[3]
B	150		8.82			
A	130	17	7.65	WFI	✓ (P) (24 h)	CLIN
B	150		8.82			
A	20	2	10.00	WFI	✓ (P) (24 h)	CLIN
B	5		2.50			
A	–	–	15.00	WFI	✓ (PC) (24 h)	LAB[5]
B	–		15.00			
A	300	15	20.00	WFI	✓ (PC) (24 h)	LAB[4]
B	100		6.67			
A	200	10	20.00	WFI	✓ (PC) (24 h)	LAB[4]
B	100		10.00			
A	50	2	25.00	WFI	✓ (PC) (24 h)	LAB[3]
B	5		2.50			
A	250	10	25.00	WFI	☒ (SEE ABOVE)	LAB[4]
B	100		10.00			
A	450	17	26.47	WFI	✓ (P) (24 h)	CLIN
B	150		8.82			
A	550	17	32.35	WFI	✓ (P) (24 h)	CLIN
B	150		8.82			
A	–	–	37.5	WFI	☒ (SEE ABOVE)	LAB[5]
B	–		12.5			
A	100	2	50.00	WFI	✓ (PC) (24 h)	LAB[3]
B	5		2.5			
A	840	9.5	88.42	WFI	☒ (SEE ABOVE)	CLIN
B	150		15.79			

Diamorphine (A) and Dexamethasone (B)

Summary: No problems with physical stability encountered, although precipitation/turbidity may occur as dexamethasone dose increases. Note that diamorphine degradation increases as the pH increases (see page 42). Dexamethasone is usually given as a sub-cutaneous bolus injection (depending upon volume of injection) or via a separate CSCI. However, if dexamethasone is to be mixed with other drugs, it should be the last constituent added to the maximally diluted syringe. There may be initial transient turbidity upon the addition of dexamethasone.

Drug	Dose in syringe (mg)	Volume in syringe (ml)	Concentration (mg/ml)	Diluent	Outcome	Data Type
A	15	17	0.88	WFI	✓ (P) (24 h)	CLIN
B	16		0.94			
A	50	16	3.13	WFI	✓ (P) (24 h)	CLIN
B	12		0.75			
A	70	17	4.12	WFI	✓ (P) (24 h)	CLIN
B	8		0.47			

Diamorphine (A) and Haloperidol (B)

Summary: Mixture may be incompatible at high concentrations.

Drug	Dose in syringe (mg)	Volume in syringe (ml)	Concentration (mg/ml)	Diluent	Outcome	Data Type
A	30	17	1.76	WFI	✓ (P) (24 h)	CLIN
B	5		0.29			
A	20	10	2.00	WFI	✓ (PC) (> 24 h)	LAB³
B	7.5		0.75			
A	45	17	2.65	WFI	✓ (P) (24 h)	CLIN
B	10		0.59			
A	80	17	4.71	WFI	✓ (P) (24 h)	CLIN
B	15		0.88			
A	300	15	20.00	WFI	✓ (P) (24 h)	CLIN
B	10		0.67			
A	200	10	20.00	WFI	✓ (PC) (> 24 h)	LAB³
B	7.5		0.75			
A	430	15	28.67	WFI	✓ (P) (24 h)	CLIN
B	15		1.00			
A	500	17	29.41	WFI	✓ (P) (24 h)	CLIN
B	10		0.59			
A	50	1	50.00	WFI	✓ (P) (7 days)	LAB⁴
B	4		4.00			
A	–	–	50.00	–	☒	LAB⁵
B	–		5.00			
A	100	1	100.00	WFI	✓ (P) (7 days)	LAB⁴
B	2		2.00			
A	100	1	100.00	WFI	✓ (P) (7 days)	LAB⁴
B	3		3.00			

Diamorphine (A) and Hyoscine Butylbromide (B)

Summary: No problems with physical stability encountered.

Drug	Dose in syringe (mg)	Volume in syringe (ml)	Concentration (mg/ml)	Diluent	Outcome	Data Type
A	20	17	1.18	WFI	✓ (P) (24 h)	CLIN
B	60		3.53			
A	30	17	1.76	WFI	✓ (P) (24 h)	CLIN
B	80		4.71			
A	70	17	4.12	WFI	✓ (P) (24 h)	CLIN
B	80		4.71			
A	100	17	5.88	WFI	✓ (P) (24 h)	CLIN
B	120		7.06			
A	–	–	50.00	–	✓ (PC) (24 h)	LAB[5]
B	–		20.00			
A	–	–	150.00	–	✓ (PC) (24 h)	LAB[5]
B	–		20.00			

Diamorphine (A) and Hyoscine Hydrobromide (B)

Summary: No problems with physical stability encountered.

Drug	Dose in syringe (mg)	Volume in syringe (ml)	Concentration (mg/ml)	Diluent	Outcome	Data Type
A	–	–	50.00	–	✓ (PC) (24 h)	LAB[5]
B	–		0.4			
A	–	–	150.00	–	✓ (PC) (24 h)	LAB[5]
B	–		0.4			

Diamorphine (A) and Ketorolac (B)

Summary: No problems with physical stability encountered. However, chemical and physical incompatibilities may occur as concentrations change.

Drug	Dose in syringe (mg)	Volume in syringe (ml)	Concentration (mg/ml)	Diluent	Outcome	Data Type
A	50	8.5	5.88	NaCl	✓ (P) (24 h)	CLIN
B	90		10.59			
A	4000	20	200.00	–	✓ (P) (24 h)	LAB[6]
B	120		6.00			

Diamorphine (A) and Levomepromazine (B)

Summary: No problems with physical stability encountered. To avoid irritation at the site of infusion, levomepromazine may be given as a subcutaneous bolus injection at doses below 50 mg (= 2 ml).

Drug	Dose in syringe (mg)	Volume in syringe (ml)	Concentration (mg/ml)	Diluent	Outcome	Data Type
A	50	17	2.94	WFI	✓ (P) (24 h)	CLIN
B	18.75		1.10			
A	150	17	8.82	WFI	✓ (P) (24 h)	CLIN
B	25		1.47			
A	80	9	8.89	WFI	✓ (P) (24 h)	CLIN
B	37.5		4.17			
A	180	17	10.59	NaCl	✓ (P) (24 h)	CLIN
B	25		1.47			
A	200	17	11.76	WFI	✓ (P) (24 h)	CLIN
B	25		1.47			
A	200	17	11.76	WFI	✓ (P) (24 h)	CLIN
B	50		2.94			
A	180	10	18.00	WFI	✓ (P) (24 h)	CLIN
B	25		2.50			

Diamorphine (A) and Metoclopramide (B)

Summary: No problems with physical stability encountered.

Drug	Dose in syringe (mg)	Volume in syringe (ml)	Concentration (mg/ml)	Diluent	Outcome	Data Type
A	20	21	0.95	NaCl	✓ (P) (24 h)	CLIN
B	100		4.76			
A	40	17	2.35	WFI	✓ (P) (24 h)	CLIN
B	30		1.76			
A	50	17	2.94	WFI	✓ (P) (24 h)	CLIN
B	40		2.35			
A	150	17	8.82	WFI	✓ (P) (24 h)	CLIN
B	60		3.53			
A	350	10	35.00	WFI	✓ (P) (24 h)	CLIN
B	30		3.00			
A	–	–	50.00	–	✓ (P) (24 h)	LAB[5]
B	–		5.00			
A	–	–	150.00	–	✓ (P) (24 h)	LAB[5]
B	–		5.00			

Diamorphine (A) and Midazolam (B)

Summary: No problems with physical stability encountered.

Drug	Dose in syringe (mg)	Volume in syringe (ml)	Concentration (mg/ml)	Diluent	Outcome	Data Type
A	10	17	0.59	WFI	✓ (P) (24 h)	CLIN
B	10		0.59			
A	50	17	2.94	WFI	✓ (P) (24 h)	CLIN
B	20		1.18			
A	180	17	10.59	WFI	✓ (P) (24 h)	CLIN
B	40		2.35			
A	320	15	21.33	WFI	✓ (P) (24 h)	CLIN
B	60		4.00			
A	450	17	26.47	WFI	✓ (P) (24 h)	CLIN
B	25		1.47			
A	1400	17	82.35	WFI	✓ (P) (24 h)	CLIN
B	30		1.76			
A	2300**	15	153.33	WFI	✓ (P) (24 h)	CLIN
B	30		2.00			

**Reconstituted with 2 ml diluent.

Diamorphine (A) and Octreotide (B)

Summary: No problems with physical stability encountered.

Drug	Dose in syringe (mg)	Volume in syringe (ml)	Concentration (mg/ml)	Diluent	Outcome	Data Type
A	120	17	7.06	WFI	✔ (P) (24 h)	CLIN
B	0.6		0.04			
A	50	8	6.25	WFI	✔ (PC) (24 h)	LAB [7]
B	0.3		0.04			
A	50	8	6.25	WFI	✔ (PC) (24 h)	LAB [7]
B	0.6		0.08			
A	50	8	6.25	WFI	✔ (PC) (24 h)	LAB [7]
B	0.9		0.11			
A	100	8	12.50	WFI	✔ (PC) (24 h)	LAB [7]
B	0.3		0.04			
A	100	8	12.50	WFI	✔ (PC) (24 h)	LAB [7]
B	0.6		0.08			
A	100	8	12.50	WFI	✔ (PC) (24 h)	LAB [7]
B	0.9		0.11			
A	280	17	16.47	WFI	✔ (P) (24 h)	CLIN
B	0.6		0.04			
A	200	8	25.00	WFI	✔ (PC) (24 h)	LAB [7]
B	0.6		0.08			

Diamorphine (A) and Ondansetron (B)

Summary: No problems with physical stability encountered.

Drug	Dose in syringe (mg)	Volume in syringe (ml)	Concentration (mg/ml)	Diluent	Outcome	Data Type
A	720	17	42.35	WFI	✔ (P) (24 h)	CLIN
B	24		1.41			

Dihydrocodeine (A) and Cyclizine (B)

Summary: No problems with physical stability encountered.

Drug	Dose in syringe (mg)	Volume in syringe (ml)	Concentration (mg/ml)	Diluent	Outcome	Data Type
A	150	20	7.50	WFI	✓ (P) (24 h)	LAB
B	150		7.50			

Dihydrocodeine (A) and Dexamethasone (B)

Summary: No problems with physical stability encountered. Dexamethasone is usually given as a subcutaneous bolus injection (depending upon volume of injection) or via a separate CSCI. However, if dexamethasone is to be mixed with other drugs, it should be the last constituent added to the maximally diluted syringe. There may be initial transient turbidity upon the addition of dexamethasone.

Drug	Dose in syringe (mg)	Volume in syringe (ml)	Concentration (mg/ml)	Diluent	Outcome	Data Type
A	150	20	7.50	WFI	✓ (P) (24 h)	LAB
B	16		0.80			

Dihydrocodeine (A) and Haloperidol (B)

Summary: No problems with physical stability encountered.

Drug	Dose in syringe (mg)	Volume in syringe (ml)	Concentration (mg/ml)	Diluent	Outcome	Data Type
A	150	20	7.50	WFI	✓ (P) (24 h)	LAB
B	15		0.75			

Dihydrocodeine (A) and Levomepromazine (B)

Summary: No problems with physical stability encountered. To avoid irritation at the site of infusion, levomepromazine may be given as a subcutaneous bolus injection at doses below 50 mg (= 2 ml).

Drug	Dose in syringe (mg)	Volume in syringe (ml)	Concentration (mg/ml)	Diluent	Outcome	Data Type
A	150	20	7.50	WFI	✓ (P) (24 h)	LAB
B	50		2.50			

Fentanyl (A) and Dexamethasone (B)

Summary: No problems with physical stability encountered.

Drug	Dose in syringe (mg)	Volume in syringe (ml)	Concentration (mg/ml)	Diluent	Outcome	Data Type
A	0.125	10	0.01	DEX	✓ (PC) (24 h)	LAB[8]
B	5		0.50			

Fentanyl (A) and Haloperidol (B)

Summary: No problems with physical stability encountered.

Drug	Dose in syringe (mg)	Volume in syringe (ml)	Concentration (mg/ml)	Diluent	Outcome	Data Type
A	0.125	10	0.01	DEX	✓ (PC) (24 h)	LAB[8]
B	5		0.10			

Fentanyl (A) and Hyoscine Hydrobromide (B)

Summary: No problems with physical stability encountered.

Drug	Dose in syringe (mg)	Volume in syringe (ml)	Concentration (mg/ml)	Diluent	Outcome	Data Type
A	0.125	10	0.01	DEX	✓ (PC) (24 h)	LAB[8]
B	0.25		0.03			

Fentanyl (A) and Ketamine (B)

Summary: No problems with physical stability encountered.

Drug	Dose in syringe (mg)	Volume in syringe (ml)	Concentration (mg/ml)	Diluent	Outcome	Data Type
A	0.125	10	0.01	DEX	✔ (PC) (24 h)	LAB[8]
B	5.0		0.50			

Fentanyl (A) and Levomepromazine (B)

Summary: No problems with physical stability encountered.

Drug	Dose in syringe (mg)	Volume in syringe (ml)	Concentration (mg/ml)	Diluent	Outcome	Data Type
A	0.125	10	0.01	DEX	✔ (PC) (24 h)	LAB[8]
B	5.0		0.10			

Fentanyl (A) and Metoclopramide (B)

Summary: No problems with physical stability encountered.

Drug	Dose in syringe (mg)	Volume in syringe (ml)	Concentration (mg/ml)	Diluent	Outcome	Data Type
A	0.125	10	0.01	DEX	✔ (PC) (24 h)	LAB[8]
B	25		2.50			

Fentanyl (A) and Midazolam (B)

Summary: No problems with physical stability encountered.

Drug	Dose in syringe (mg)	Volume in syringe (ml)	Concentration (mg/ml)	Diluent	Outcome	Data Type
A	0.125	10	0.01	DEX	✓ (PC) (24 h)	LAB[8]
B	1.0		0.10			
A	0.1	8	0.01	NaCl	✓ (PC) (24 h)	LAB[9]
B	5		0.63			
A	0.1	8	0.01	NaCl	✓ (PC) (24 h)	LAB[9]
B	7.5		0.94			
A	0.3	8	0.04	NaCl	✓ (PC) (24 h)	LAB[9]
B	5		0.63			
A	0.3	8	0.04	NaCl	✓ (PC) (24 h)	LAB[9]
B	7.5		0.94			
A	0.6	18	0.03	NaCl	✓ (PC) (24 h)	LAB[9]
B	15		0.83			
A	0.6	18	0.03	NaCl	✓ (PC) (24 h)	LAB[9]
B	5		0.28			

Fentanyl (A) and Ondansetron (B)

Summary: No problems with physical stability encountered.

Drug	Dose in syringe (mg)	Volume in syringe (ml)	Concentration (mg/ml)	Diluent	Outcome	Data Type
A	0.585	35	0.02	NaCl	✓ (PC) (24 h)	LAB[2]
B	46.5		1.33			

Hydromorphone (A) and Dimenhydrinate (B)

Summary: No problems with physical stability encountered.

Drug	Dose in syringe (mg)	Volume in syringe (ml)	Concentration (mg/ml)	Diluent	Outcome	Data Type
A	2	2	1.00	WFI	✓ (P)	LAB[10]
B	50		25.00		(24 h)	
A	10	2	5.00	WFI	✓ (P)	LAB[10]
B	50		25.00		(24 h)	
A	40	2	20.00	WFI	✓ (P)	LAB[10]
B	50		25.00		(24 h)	

Hydromorphone (A) and Haloperidol (B)

Summary: No problems with physical stability encountered.

Drug	Dose in syringe (mg)	Volume in syringe (ml)	Concentration (mg/ml)	Diluent	Outcome	Data Type
A	40	18	2.22	NaCl	✓ (P)	CLIN
B	1		0.06		(24 h)	
A	50	18	2.78	NaCl	✓ (P)	CLIN
B	1		0.06		(24 h)	

Hydromorphone (A) and Midazolam (B)

Summary: No problems with physical stability encountered.

Drug	Dose in syringe (mg)	Volume in syringe (ml)	Concentration (mg/ml)	Diluent	Outcome	Data Type
A	18	18	1.00	NaCl	✓ (P)	CLIN
B	5		0.28		(24 h)	
A	30	18	1.67	NaCl	✓ (P)	CLIN
B	10		0.56		(24 h)	

Methadone (A) and Clonazepam (B)

Summary: No problems with physical stability encountered. Loss of clonazepam observed when infused via PVC tubing.[1] Minimize loss by using non-PVC tubing.

Drug	Dose in syringe (mg)	Volume in syringe (ml)	Concentration (mg/ml)	Diluent	Outcome	Data Type
A	60	17	3.53	NaCl	✓ (P) (24 h)	CLIN
B	2		0.12			

Methadone (A) and Midazolam (B)

Summary: No problems with physical stability encountered.

Drug	Dose in syringe (mg)	Volume in syringe (ml)	Concentration (mg/ml)	Diluent	Outcome	Data Type
A	25	16	1.56	NaCl	✓ (P) (24 h)	CLIN
B	20		1.25			

Morphine Hydrochloride (A) and Dexamethasone (B)

Summary: No problems with physical stability encountered. Dexamethasone is usually given as a subcutaneous bolus injection (depending upon volume of injection) or via a separate CSCI. However, if dexamethasone is to be mixed with other drugs, it should be the last constituent added to the maximally diluted syringe. There may be initial transient turbidity upon the addition of dexamethasone.

Drug	Dose in syringe (mg)	Volume in syringe (ml)	Concentration (mg/ml)	Diluent	Outcome	Data Type
A	300	60	5.00	NaCl	✓ (P) (5 days)†	LAB[11]
B	80		1.33			

†Infusion rate set at 0.5 ml/hour over the 5 days.

Morphine Hydrochloride (A) and Haloperidol (B)

Summary: No problems with physical stability encountered.

Drug	Dose in syringe (mg)	Volume in syringe (ml)	Concentration (mg/ml)	Diluent	Outcome	Data Type
A	300	60	5.00	NaCl	✓ (P)	LAB[11]
B	3.75		0.63		(5 days)[†]	

[†]Infusion rate set at 0.5 ml/hour over the 5 days.

Morphine Hydrochloride (A) and Hyoscine Butylbromide (B)

Summary: No problems with physical stability encountered.

Drug	Dose in syringe (mg)	Volume in syringe (ml)	Concentration (mg/ml)	Diluent	Outcome	Data Type
A	300	60	5.00	NaCl	✓ (P)	LAB[11]
B	300		5.00		(5 days)[†]	

[†]Infusion rate set at 0.5 ml/hour over the 5 days.

Morphine Hydrochloride (A) and Metoclopramide (B)

Summary: No problems with physical stability encountered.

Drug	Dose in syringe (mg)	Volume in syringe (ml)	Concentration (mg/ml)	Diluent	Outcome	Data Type
A	300	60	5.00	NaCl	✓ (P)	LAB[11]
B	200		3.33		(5 days)[†]	

[†]Infusion rate set at 0.5 ml/hour over the 5 days.

Morphine Hydrochloride (A) and Midazolam (B)

Summary: No problems with physical stability encountered.

Drug	Dose in syringe (mg)	Volume in syringe (ml)	Concentration (mg/ml)	Diluent	Outcome	Data Type
A	300	60	5.00	NaCl	✓ (P)	LAB[11]
B	90		1.50		(5 days)[†]	

[†]Infusion rate set at 0.5 ml/hour over the 5 days.

Morphine Sulphate (A) and Cyclizine (B)

Summary: No problems with physical stability encountered.

Drug	Dose in syringe (mg)	Volume in syringe (ml)	Concentration (mg/ml)	Diluent	Outcome	Data Type
A	10	18	0.56	WFI	✓ (P) (24 h)	CLIN
B	100		5.56			
A	15	18	0.83	WFI	✓ (P) (24 h)	CLIN
B	100		5.56			
A	15	8	1.88	WFI	✓ (P) (24 h)	CLIN
B	100		12.50			

Morphine Sulphate (A) and Haloperidol (B)

Summary: No problems with physical stability encountered.

Drug	Dose in syringe (mg)	Volume in syringe (ml)	Concentration (mg/ml)	Diluent	Outcome	Data Type
A	10	18	0.56	NaCl	✓ (P) (24 h)	CLIN
B	1		0.06			
A	10	18	0.56	NaCl	✓ (P) (24 h)	CLIN
B	12		0.67			
A	10	8	1.25	NaCl	✓ (P) (24 h)	CLIN
B	1		0.13			
A	40	18	2.22	NaCl	✓ (P) (24 h)	CLIN
B	5		0.28			
A	20	8	2.50	NaCl	✓ (P) (24 h)	CLIN
B	1		0.13			
A	60	18	3.33	NaCl	✓ (P) (24 h)	CLIN
B	2		0.11			
A	30	8	3.75	NaCl	✓ (P) (24 h)	CLIN
B	0.5		0.06			
A	70	18	3.89	NaCl	✓ (P) (24 h)	CLIN
B	5		0.28			
A	50	18	2.78	NaCl	✓ (P) (24 h)	CLIN
B	5		0.28			
A	60	8	7.50	NaCl	✓ (P) (24 h)	CLIN
B	4		0.5			

Morphine Sulphate (A) and Metoclopramide (B)

Summary: No problems with physical stability encountered.

Drug	Dose in syringe (mg)	Volume in syringe (ml)	Concentration (mg/ml)	Diluent	Outcome	Data Type
A	5	8	0.63	NaCl	✓ (P)	CLIN
B	30		3.75		(24 h)	
A	30	18	1.67	NaCl	✓ (P)	CLIN
B	20		1.11		(24 h)	

Morphine Sulphate (A) and Ondansetron (B)

Summary: No problems with physical stability encountered.

Drug	Dose in syringe (mg)	Volume in syringe (ml)	Concentration (mg/ml)	Diluent	Outcome	Data Type
A	93.3	35	2.67	NaCl	✓ (P)	LAB[2]
B	46.6		1.33		(24 h)	

Morphine Tartrate (A) and Dexamethasone (B)

Summary: No problems with physical stability encountered. Dexamethasone is usually given as a subcutaneous bolus injection (depending upon volume of injection) or via a separate CSCI. However, if dexamethasone is to be mixed with other drugs, it should be the last constituent added to the maximally diluted syringe. There may be initial transient turbidity upon the addition of dexamethasone.

Drug	Dose in syringe (mg)	Volume in syringe (ml)	Concentration (mg/ml)	Diluent	Outcome	Data Type
A	100	18	5.56	NaCl	✓ (P)	CLIN
B	2		0.11		(24 h)	
A	720	18	40.00	NaCl	✓ (P)	CLIN
B	8		0.44		(24 h)	

Morphine Tartrate (A) and Haloperidol (B)

Summary: No problems with physical stability encountered.

Drug	Dose in syringe (mg)	Volume in syringe (ml)	Concentration (mg/ml)	Diluent	Outcome	Data Type
A	180	18	10.00	NaCl	✓ (P) (24 h)	CLIN
B	5		0.28			

Morphine Tartrate (A) and Metoclopramide (B)

Summary: No problems with physical stability encountered.

Drug	Dose in syringe (mg)	Volume in syringe (ml)	Concentration (mg/ml)	Diluent	Outcome	Data Type
A	100	18	5.56	NaCl	✓ (P) (24 h)	CLIN
B	10		0.56			
A	420	18	23.33	NaCl	✓ (P) (24 h)	CLIN
B	30		1.67			
A	480	18	26.67	NaCl	✓ (P) (24 h)	CLIN
B	30		1.67			

Oxycodone (A) and Clonazepam (B)

Summary: No problems with physical stability encountered. Loss of clonazepam observed when infused via PVC tubing.[1] Minimize loss by using non-PVC tubing.

Drug	Dose in syringe (mg)	Volume in syringe (ml)	Concentration (mg/ml)	Diluent	Outcome	Data Type
A	100	20	5.00	WFI	✓ (P) (24 h)	LAB[12]
B	4		0.20			
A	100	20	5.00	NaCl	✓ (P) (24 h)	LAB[12]
B	4		0.20			

Oxycodone (A) and Cyclizine (B)

Summary: Problems with physical compatibility are likely as concentrations of either drug increase (compare diamorphine/cyclizine)

Drug	Dose in syringe (mg)	Volume in syringe (ml)	Concentration (mg/ml)	Diluent	Outcome	Data Type
A	20	20.4	0.98	WFI	✓ (P) (24 h)	LAB[13]
B	20		0.98			
A	50	19	2.63	WFI	✓ (P) (24 h)	LAB[13]
B	150		7.89			
A	200	22	9.09	–	✓ (P) (24 h)	LAB[13]
B	100		4.55			
A	200	23	8.70	–	✗	LAB[13]
B	150		6.52			

Oxycodone (A) and Dexamethasone (B)

Summary: No problems with physical stability encountered. Dexamethasone is usually given as a subcutaneous bolus injection (depending upon volume of injection) or via a separate CSCI. However, if dexamethasone is to be mixed with other drugs, it should be the last constituent added to the maximally diluted syringe. There may be initial transient turbidity upon the addition of dexamethasone.

Drug	Dose in syringe (mg)	Volume in syringe (ml)	Concentration (mg/ml)	Diluent	Outcome	Data Type
A	20	25	0.80	WFI	✓ (PC) (24 h)	LAB[13]
B	20		0.80			
A	20	25	0.80	NaCl	✓ (PC) (24 h)	LAB[13]
B	20		0.80			
A	200	30	6.67	–	✓ (PC) (24 h)	LAB[13]
B	40		1.33			

Oxycodone (A) and Haloperidol (B)

Summary: No problems with physical stability encountered.

Drug	Dose in syringe (mg)	Volume in syringe (ml)	Concentration (mg/ml)	Diluent	Outcome	Data Type
A	20	20.5	0.98	WFI	✓ (PC) (24 h)	LAB[13]
B	2.5		0.12			
A	20	20.5	0.98	NaCl	✓ (PC) (24 h)	LAB[13]
B	2.5		0.12			
A	200	23	8.70	–	✓ (PC) (24 h)	LAB[13]
B	15		0.65			

Oxycodone (A) and Hyoscine Butylbromide (B)

Summary: No problems with physical stability encountered.

Drug	Dose in syringe (mg)	Volume in syringe (ml)	Concentration (mg/ml)	Diluent	Outcome	Data Type
A	20	21	0.95	WFI	✓ (PC) (24 h)	LAB[13]
B	20		0.95			
A	20	21	0.95	NaCl	✓ (PC) (24 h)	LAB[13]
B	20		0.95			
A	200	23	8.70	–	✓ (PC) (24 h)	LAB[13]
B	60		2.61			

Oxycodone (A) and Hyoscine Hydrobromide (B)

Summary: No problems with physical stability encountered.

Drug	Dose in syringe (mg)	Volume in syringe (ml)	Concentration (mg/ml)	Diluent	Outcome	Data Type
A	20	21.5	0.93	WFI	✓ (PC) (24 h)	LAB[13]
B	0.6		0.03			
A	20	21.5	0.93	NaCl	✓ (PC) (24 h)	LAB[13]
B	0.6		0.03			
A	200	26	7.69	–	✓ (PC) (24 h)	LAB[13]
B	2.4		0.09			

Oxycodone (A) and Ketamine (B)

Summary: No problems with physical stability encountered.

Drug	Dose in syringe (mg)	Volume in syringe (ml)	Concentration (mg/ml)	Diluent	Outcome	Data Type
A	100	20	5.00	NaCl	✓ (P) (24 h)	LAB[12]
B	300		15.00			

Oxycodone (A) and Ketorolac (B)

Summary: No problems with physical stability encountered.

Drug	Dose in syringe (mg)	Volume in syringe (ml)	Concentration (mg/ml)	Diluent	Outcome	Data Type
A	100	20	5.00	NaCl	✓ (P) (24 h)	LAB[12]
B	90		4.50			

Oxycodone (A) and Levomepromazine (B)

Summary: No problems with physical stability encountered. To reduce irritation at the site of infusion, levomepromazine may be given as a subcutaneous bolus injection at doses below 50 mg (= 2 ml).

Drug	Dose in syringe (mg)	Volume in syringe (ml)	Concentration (mg/ml)	Diluent	Outcome	Data Type
A	20	20.2	0.99	WFI	✓ (PC) (24 h)	LAB[13]
B	5		0.25			
A	20	20.2	0.99	NaCl	✓ (PC) (24 h)	LAB[13]
B	5		0.25			
A	200	28	7.14	–	✓ (PC) (24 h)	LAB[13]
B	200		7.14			

Oxycodone (A) and Metoclopramide (B)

Summary: No problems with physical stability encountered.

Drug	Dose in syringe (mg)	Volume in syringe (ml)	Concentration (mg/ml)	Diluent	Outcome	Data Type
A	20	26	0.77	WFI	✓ (PC) (24 h)	LAB[13]
B	30		1.15			
A	20	26	0.77	NaCl	✓ (PC) (24 h)	LAB[13]
B	30		1.15			
A	200	40	5.00	–	✓ (PC) (24 h)	LAB[13]
B	100		2.50			

Oxycodone (A) and Midazolam (B)

Summary: No problems with physical stability encountered.

Drug	Dose in syringe (mg)	Volume in syringe (ml)	Concentration (mg/ml)	Diluent	Outcome	Data Type
A	20	24	0.83	WFI	✓ (PC) (24 h)	LAB[13]
B	20		0.83			
A	20	24	0.83	NaCl	✓ (PC) (24 h)	LAB[13]
B	20		0.83			
A	200	40	5.00	–	✓ (PC) (24 h)	LAB[13]
B	100		2.50			

Oxycodone (A) and Octreotide (B)

Summary: No problems with physical stability encountered.

Drug	Dose in syringe (mg)	Volume in syringe (ml)	Concentration (mg/ml)	Diluent	Outcome	Data Type
A	100	20	5.00	NaCl	✓ (P) (24 h)	LAB[12]
B	0.5		0.03			

Oxycodone (A) and Ondansetron (B)

Summary: No problems with physical stability encountered.

Drug	Dose in syringe (mg)	Volume in syringe (ml)	Concentration (mg/ml)	Diluent	Outcome	Data Type
A	100	20	5.00	NaCl	✔ (P) (24 h)	LAB[12]
B	16		0.80			

Oxycodone (A) and Ranitidine (B)

Summary: No problems with physical stability encountered.

Drug	Dose in syringe (mg)	Volume in syringe (ml)	Concentration (mg/ml)	Diluent	Outcome	Data Type
A	100	20	5.00	NaCl	✔ (P) (24 h)	LAB[12]
B	150		7.50			
A	100	20	5.00	WFI	✔ (P) (24 h)	LAB[12]
B	150		7.50			

Tramadol (A) and Dexamethasone (B)

Summary: No problems with physical stability encountered. Dexamethasone is usually given as a subcutaneous bolus injection (depending upon volume of injection) or via a separate CSCI. However, if dexamethasone is to be mixed with other drugs, it should be the last constituent added to the maximally diluted syringe. There may be initial transient turbidity upon the addition of dexamethasone.

Drug	Dose in syringe (mg)	Volume in syringe (ml)	Concentration (mg/ml)	Diluent	Outcome	Data Type
A	2000	60	33.33	NaCl	✔ (P) (5 days)†	LAB[11]
B	80		1.33			

†Infusion rate set at 0.5 ml/hour over the 5 days.

Tramadol (A) and Haloperidol (B)

Summary: No problems with physical stability encountered.

Drug	Dose in syringe (mg)	Volume in syringe (ml)	Concentration (mg/ml)	Diluent	Outcome	Data Type
A	200	17	11.76	WFI	✓ (P) (24 h)	CLIN
B	10		0.59			
A	300	17	17.65	WFI	✓ (P) (24 h)	CLIN
B	5		0.29			
A	2000	60	33.33	NaCl	✓ (P) (5 days)†	LAB[11]
B	37.5		0.63			

†Infusion rate set at 0.5 ml/hour over the 5 days.

Tramadol (A) and Hyoscine Butylbromide (B)

Summary: No problems with physical stability encountered.

Drug	Dose in syringe (mg)	Volume in syringe (ml)	Concentration (mg/ml)	Diluent	Outcome	Data Type
A	2000	60	33.33	NaCl	✓ (P) (5 days)†	LAB[11]
B	300		5.00			

†Infusion rate set at 0.5 ml/hour over the 5 days.

Tramadol (A) and Metoclopramide (B)

Summary: No problems with physical stability encountered.

Drug	Dose in syringe (mg)	Volume in syringe (ml)	Concentration (mg/ml)	Diluent	Outcome	Data Type
A	2000	60	33.33	NaCl	✓ (P) (5 days)†	LAB[11]
B	200		3.33			

†Infusion rate set at 0.5 ml/hour over the 5 days.

Tramadol (A) and Midazolam (B)

Summary: No problems with physical stability encountered.

Drug	Dose in syringe (mg)	Volume in syringe (ml)	Concentration (mg/ml)	Diluent	Outcome	Data Type
A	2000	60	33.33	NaCl	✓ (P) (5 days)†	LAB[11]
B	90		1.50			

†Infusion rate set at 0.5 ml/hour over the 5 days.

Clonazepam (A) and Dexamethasone (B)

Summary: No problems with physical stability encountered. Loss of clonazepam has been observed when infused via PVC tubing. If problematic, this loss can be minimized by using non-PVC tubing.[1] Dexamethasone is usually given as a subcutaneous bolus injection (depending upon volume of injection) or via a separate CSCI. However, if dexamethasone is to be mixed with other drugs, it should be the last constituent added to the maximally diluted syringe. There may be initial transient turbidity upon the addition of dexamethasone.

Drug	Dose in syringe (mg)	Volume in syringe (ml)	Concentration (mg/ml)	Diluent	Outcome	Data Type
A	2	17	0.12	WFI	✓ (P) (24 h)	CLIN
B	16		0.94			
A	6	17	0.35	WFI	✓ (P) (24 h)	CLIN
B	6		0.35			

Clonazepam (A) and Glycopyrronium (B)

Summary: No problems with physical stability encountered. Loss of clonazepam observed when infused via PVC tubing.[1] Minimize loss by using non-PVC tubing.

Drug	Dose in syringe (mg)	Volume in syringe (ml)	Concentration (mg/ml)	Diluent	Outcome	Data Type
A	4	17	0.24	WFI	✓ (P) (24 h)	CLIN
B	1.2		0.07			

Clonazepam (A) and Haloperidol (B)

Summary: No problems with physical stability encountered. Loss of clonazepam observed when infused via PVC tubing.[1] Minimize loss by using non-PVC tubing.

Drug	Dose in syringe (mg)	Volume in syringe (ml)	Concentration (mg/ml)	Diluent	Outcome	Data Type
A	2	16	0.13	WFI	✓ (P) (24 h)	CLIN
B	5		0.31			

Clonazepam (A) and Metoclopramide (B)

Summary: No problems with physical stability encountered. Loss of clonazepam observed when infused via PVC tubing.[1] Minimize loss by using non-PVC tubing.

Drug	Dose in syringe (mg)	Volume in syringe (ml)	Concentration (mg/ml)	Diluent	Outcome	Data Type
A	2	18	0.11	NaCl	✓ (P) (24 h)	CLIN
B	20		1.11			
A	3	18	0.17	NaCl	✓ (P) (24 h)	CLIN
B	20		1.11			

Cyclizine (A) and Dexamethasone (B)

Summary: Mixture may exhibit concentration-dependent physical incompatibility. Dexamethasone is usually given as a subcutaneous bolus injection (depending upon volume of injection) or via a separate CSCI. However, if dexamethasone is to be mixed with other drugs, it should be the last constituent added to the maximally diluted syringe. There may be initial transient turbidity upon the addition of dexamethasone.

Drug	Dose in syringe (mg)	Volume in syringe (ml)	Concentration (mg/ml)	Diluent	Outcome	Data Type
A	50	6	8.33	WFI	✓ (P) (24 h)	CLIN
B	2		0.33			

Cyclizine (A) and Haloperidol (B)

Summary: No problems with physical stability encountered.

Drug	Dose in syringe (mg)	Volume in syringe (ml)	Concentration (mg/ml)	Diluent	Outcome	Data Type
A	150	17	8.82	WFI	✓ (P) (24 h)	CLIN
B	10		0.59			

Cyclizine (A) and Metoclopramide (B)

Summary: Crystallization may occur as dose of metoclopramide increases relative to cyclizine. This is NOT a sensible combination of antiemetics, since the pro-kinetic action of metoclopramide is (theoretically) inhibited by cyclizine. Higher doses of metoclopramide will be required to overcome this. However, use of this combination is acceptable if metoclopramide is used for its central dopamine antagonist properties, although haloperidol is preferable.

Drug	Dose in syringe (mg)	Volume in syringe (ml)	Concentration (mg/ml)	Diluent	Outcome	Data Type
A	150	17	8.82	WFI	✓(P) (24 h)	CLIN
B	30		1.76			
A	150	15	10.00	–	☒/✓(P) (see above)	CLIN
B	60		4.00			

Dexamethasone (A) and Haloperidol (B)

Summary: Mixture appears to exhibit concentration-dependent physical incompatibility. Dexamethasone is usually given as a subcutaneous bolus injection (depending upon volume of injection) or via a separate CSCI. However, if dexamethasone is to be mixed with other drugs, it should be the last constituent added to the maximally diluted syringe. There may be initial transient turbidity upon the addition of dexamethasone.

Drug	Dose in syringe (mg)	Volume in syringe (ml)	Concentration (mg/ml)	Diluent	Outcome	Data Type
A	2	13	0.15	NaCl	✓(P) (24 h)	LAB
B	5		0.38			
A	2	13	0.15	WFI	✓(P) (24 h)	LAB
B	5		0.38			
A	12	20	0.60	WFI	☒	LAB
B	5		0.25			
A	12	60	0.63	NaCl	☒†	LAB[11]
B	5		1.33			

†Infusion rate set at 0.5 ml/hour over the 5 days.

Dexamethasone (A) and Hyoscine Butylbromide (B)

Summary: No problems with physical stability encountered. Dexamethasone is usually given as a subcutaneous bolus injection (depending upon volume of injection) or via a separate CSCI. However, if dexamethasone is to be mixed with other drugs, it should be the last constituent added to the maximally diluted syringe. There may be initial transient turbidity upon the addition of dexamethasone.

Drug	Dose in syringe (mg)	Volume in syringe (ml)	Concentration (mg/ml)	Diluent	Outcome	Data Type
A	1	10	0.10	NaCl	✓ (P) (24 h)	CLIN
B	150		12.00			
A	1	10	0.10	WFI	✓ (P) (24 h)	CLIN
B	120		12.00			

Dexamethasone (A) and Hyoscine Hydrobromide (B)

Summary: No problems with physical stability encountered. Dexamethasone is usually given as a subcutaneous bolus injection (depending upon volume of injection) or via a separate CSCI. However, if dexamethasone is to be mixed with other drugs, it should be the last constituent added to the maximally diluted syringe. There may be initial transient turbidity upon the addition of dexamethasone.

Drug	Dose in syringe (mg)	Volume in syringe (ml)	Concentration (mg/ml)	Diluent	Outcome	Data Type
A	1	10	0.10	NaCl	✓ (P) (24 h)	CLIN
B	1.2		0.12			
A	1	10	0.10	WFI	✓ (P) (24 h)	CLIN
B	1.2		0.12			

Dexamethasone (A) and Levomepromazine (B)

Summary: Mixture appears to exhibit concentration-dependent physical incompatibility. Dexamethasone is usually given as a sub-cutaneous bolus injection (depending upon volume of injection) or via a separate CSCI. However, if dexamethasone is to be mixed with other drugs, it should be the last constituent added to the maximally diluted syringe. There may be initial transient turbidity upon the addition of dexamethasone.

Drug	Dose in syringe (mg)	Volume in syringe (ml)	Concentration (mg/ml)	Diluent	Outcome	Data Type
A	1	9	0.11	WFI	✓ (P) (24 h)	CLIN
B	25		2.78			
A	4	14	0.29	NaCl	✗	LAB
B	25		1.79			
A	2	14	0.14	WFI	✗	LAB
B	25		1.79			
A	8	15	0.53	WFI	✗	CLIN
B	50		3.33			

Dexamethasone (A) and Metoclopramide (B)

Summary: No problems with physical stability encountered.

Drug	Dose in syringe (mg)	Volume in syringe (ml)	Concentration (mg/ml)	Diluent	Outcome	Data Type
A	2	10	0.20	WFI	✓ (P) (24 h)	CLIN
B	20		2.00			
A	2	10	0.20	NaCl	✓ (P) (24 h)	CLIN
B	20		2.00			

Dexamethasone (A) and Midazolam (B)

Summary: Mixture appears to exhibit concentration-dependent physical incompatibility. Dexamethasone is usually given as a subcutaneous bolus injection (depending upon volume of injection) or via a separate CSCI. However, if dexamethasone is to be mixed with other drugs, it should be the last constituent added to the maximally diluted syringe. There may be initial transient turbidity upon the addition of dexamethasone. Note that laboratory evidence suggests the possibility of loss of midazolam at a higher temperature (37° C) which may be significant in combinations of midazolam and dexamethasone.[14]

Drug	Dose in syringe (mg)	Volume in syringe (ml)	Concentration (mg/ml)	Diluent	Outcome	Data Type
A	8	15	0.53	WFI	✓ (P) (24 h)	CLIN
B	35		2.33			
A	80	60	1.33	NaCl	✗ †	LAB[11]
B	20		1.50			

†Infusion rate set at 0.5 ml/hour over the 5 days.

Dexamethasone (A) and Promethazine (B)

Summary: Mixture appears to exhibit concentration-dependent physical incompatibility. Dexamethasone is usually given as a subcutaneous bolus injection (depending upon volume of injection) or via a separate CSCI. However, if dexamethasone is to be mixed with other drugs, it should be the last constituent added to the maximally diluted syringe. There may be initial transient turbidity upon the addition of dexamethasone.

Drug	Dose in syringe (mg)	Volume in syringe (ml)	Concentration (mg/ml)	Diluent	Outcome	Data Type
A	1	22	0.05	NaCl	✓ (P) (24 h)	LAB
B	25		1.14			
A	1	16	0.06	WFI	✗	LAB
B	75		4.69			

Dimenhydrinate (A) and Glycopyrronium (B)

Summary: Incompatible at the concentrations below.

Drug	Dose in syringe (mg)	Volume in syringe (ml)	Concentration (mg/ml)	Diluent	Outcome	Data Type
A	50	3	16.67	–	☒	LAB[15]
B	0.4		0.13			
A	50	2	25.00	–	☒	LAB[15]
B	0.2		0.10			
A	100	3	33.33	–	☒	LAB[15]
B	0.2		0.07			

Glycopyrronium (A) and Ondansetron (B)

Summary: No problems with physical stability encountered.

Drug	Dose in syringe (mg)	Volume in syringe (ml)	Concentration (mg/ml)	Diluent	Outcome	Data Type
A	0.8	16.5	0.05	NaCl	✓ (P) (24 h)	CLIN
B	20		1.21			
A	1.2	16	0.08	NaCl	✓ (P) (12 h)	CLIN
B	16		1.00			
A	3.5	35	0.1	NaCl	✓ (PC) (24 h)	LAB[2]
B	35		1.00			

Glycopyrronium (A) and Ranitidine (B)

Summary: No problems with physical stability encountered.

Drug	Dose in syringe (mg)	Volume in syringe (ml)	Concentration (mg/ml)	Diluent	Outcome	Data Type
A	0.6	17	0.04	WFI	✓ (P) (24 h)	CLIN
B	150		8.82			

Haloperidol (A) and Hyoscine Butylbromide (B)

Summary: Mixture exhibits concentration-dependent physical incompatibility, although problems are unlikely at usual clinical doses.

Drug	Dose in syringe (mg)	Volume in syringe (ml)	Concentration (mg/ml)	Diluent	Outcome	Data Type
A	5	15	0.33	WFI	✓ (P) (24 h)	CLIN
B	80		5.33			
A	37.5	60	0.63	NaCl	✓ (P) (5 days)†	LAB[11]
B	300		5.00			
A	75	60	1.25	NaCl	✗	LAB[16]
B	600		10.00			

†Infusion rate set at 0.5 ml/hour over the 5 days.

Haloperidol (A) and Ketamine (B)

Summary: No problems with physical stability encountered.

Drug	Dose in syringe (mg)	Volume in syringe (ml)	Concentration (mg/ml)	Diluent	Outcome	Data Type
A	10	8	1.25	NaCl	✓ (P) (24 h)	CLIN
B	150		18.75			

Haloperidol (A) and Metoclopramide (B)

Summary: Although no problems with physical stability were encountered, the use of this combination is not generally recommended because of the increased risk of adverse effects.

Drug	Dose in syringe (mg)	Volume in syringe (ml)	Concentration (mg/ml)	Diluent	Outcome	Data Type
A	37.5	60	0.63	NaCl	✓ (P) (5 days)†	LAB[11]
B	200		3.33			

†Infusion rate set at 0.5 ml/hour over the 5 days.

Haloperidol (A) and Midazolam (B)

Summary: No problems with physical stability encountered.

Drug	Dose in syringe (mg)	Volume in syringe (ml)	Concentration (mg/ml)	Diluent	Outcome	Data Type
A	37.5	60	0.63	NaCl	✓ (P) (5 days)†	LAB[11]
B	90		1.50			

†Infusion rate set at 0.5 ml/hour over the 5 days.

Hyoscine Butylbromide (A) and Midazolam (B)

Summary: No problems with physical stability encountered.

Drug	Dose in syringe (mg)	Volume in syringe (ml)	Concentration (mg/ml)	Diluent	Outcome	Data Type
A	300	60	5.00	NaCl	✓ (P)	LAB[11]
B	90		1.50		(5 days)[†]	

[†]Infusion rate set at 0.5 ml/hour over the 5 days.

Ketamine (A) and Midazolam (B)

Summary: No problems with physical stability encountered.

Drug	Dose in syringe (mg)	Volume in syringe (ml)	Concentration (mg/ml)	Diluent	Outcome	Data Type
A	100	8	12.5	NaCl	✓ (P)	CLIN
B	5		0.63		(24 h)	
A	400	18	22.22	NaCl	✓ (P)	CLIN
B	2.5		0.14		(24 h)	
A	300	17	17.65	NaCl	✓ (P)	CLIN
B	30		1.79		(24 h)	
A	300	9.5	31.58	NaCl	✓ (P)	CLIN
B	20		2.11		(24 h)	

Ketorolac (A) and Ranitidine (B)

Summary: No problems with physical stability encountered.

Drug	Dose in syringe (mg)	Volume in syringe (ml)	Concentration (mg/ml)	Diluent	Outcome	Data Type
A	30	17	1.76	NaCl	✓ (P)	CLIN
B	150		8.82		(24 h)	
A	90	20	4.50	NaCl	✓ (P)	CLIN
B	150		7.50		(24 h)	

Levomepromazine (A) and Octreotide (B)

Summary: No problems with physical stability encountered. To avoid irritation at the site of infusion, levomepromazine may be given as a subcutaneous bolus injection at doses below 50 mg (= 2 ml).

Drug	Dose in syringe (mg)	Volume in syringe (ml)	Concentration (mg/ml)	Diluent	Outcome	Data Type
A	12.5	17	0.74	WFI	✓(P) (24 h)	CLIN
B	0.3		0.02			
A	25	20	1.25	WFI	✓(P) (24 h)	CLIN
B	0.5		0.03			
A	50	17	2.94	WFI	✓(P) (24 h)	CLIN
B	0.6		0.04			

Levomepromazine (A) and Ranitidine (B)

Summary: Combination appears to exhibit concentration-dependent physical incompatibility.

Drug	Dose in syringe (mg)	Volume in syringe (ml)	Concentration (mg/ml)	Diluent	Outcome	Data Type
A	12.5	17	0.74	NaCl	✓(P) (24 h)	CLIN
B	150		8.82			
A	25	16	1.56	WFI	✗	LAB
B	100		6.25			
A	25	10	2.50	NaCl	✗	LAB
B	50		5.00			
A	25	10	2.50	WFI	✗	LAB
B	50		5.00			
A	100	3	33.33	–	✗	LAB[17]
B	25		8.33			

Metoclopramide (A) and Midazolam (B)
Summary: No problems with physical stability encountered.

Drug	Dose in syringe (mg)	Volume in syringe (ml)	Concentration (mg/ml)	Diluent	Outcome	Data Type
A	200	60	3.33	NaCl	✓(P) (5 days)†	LAB[11]
B	90		1.50			

†Infusion rate set at 0.5 ml/hour over the 5 days.

Metoclopramide (A) and Octreotide (B)

Summary: No problems with physical stability encountered.

Drug	Dose in syringe (mg)	Volume in syringe (ml)	Concentration (mg/ml)	Diluent	Outcome	Data Type
A	60	17	3.53	WFI	✓ (P) (24 h)	CLIN
B	0.6		0.04			

Metoclopramide (A) and Ondansetron (B)

Summary: No problems with physical stability encountered.

Drug	Dose in syringe (mg)	Volume in syringe (ml)	Concentration (mg/ml)	Diluent	Outcome	Data Type
A	87.5	35	2.50	NaCl	✓ (P) (24 h)	LAB[2]
B	35		1.00			

Midazolam (A) and Ondansetron (B)

Summary: No problems with physical stability encountered.

Drug	Dose in syringe (mg)	Volume in syringe (ml)	Concentration (mg/ml)	Diluent	Outcome	Data Type
A	58.3	35	1.67	NaCl	✓ (P) (24 h)	LAB[2]
B	46.5		1.33			

Octreotide (A) and Ondansetron (B)

Summary: No problems with physical stability encountered.

Drug	Dose in syringe (mg)	Volume in syringe (ml)	Concentration (mg/ml)	Diluent	Outcome	Data Type
A	0.6	22	0.03	NaCl	✓ (P) (24 h)	CLIN
B	24		1.09			
A	0.6	22	0.03	WFI	✓ (P) (24 h)	CLIN
B	24		1.09			

Compatibility data tables

Three Drugs

Drug A	B	C	Page
Alfentanil	Clonazepam	Cyclizine	162
Alfentanil	Clonazepam	Glycopyrronium	162
Alfentanil	Clonazepam	Haloperidol	163
Alfentanil	Clonazepam	Hyoscine Hydrobromide	163
Alfentanil	Cyclizine	Midazolam	164
Alfentanil	Haloperidol	Midazolam	164
Alfentanil	Hyoscine Butylbromide	Levomepromazine	165
Alfentanil	Levomepromazine	Midazolam	165
Alfentanil	Levomepromazine	Octreotide	166
Alfentanil	Metoclopramide	Midazolam	166
Diamorphine	Clonazepam	Cyclizine	167
Diamorphine	Clonazepam	Dexamethasone	167
Diamorphine	Clonazepam	Glycopyrronium	168
Diamorphine	Clonazepam	Haloperidol	168
Diamorphine	Clonazepam	Hyoscine Butylbromide	169
Diamorphine	Clonazepam	Levomepromazine	169
Diamorphine	Cyclizine	Dexamethasone	170
Diamorphine	Cyclizine	Haloperidol	171
Diamorphine	Cyclizine	Hyoscine Butylbromide	172
Diamorphine	Cyclizine	Hyoscine Hydrobromide	172
Diamorphine	Cyclizine	Levomepromazine	173
Diamorphine	Cyclizine	Metoclopramide	174
Diamorphine	Cyclizine	Midazolam	175
Diamorphine	Dexamethasone	Haloperidol	176
Diamorphine	Dexamethasone	Hyoscine Hydrobromide	177
Diamorphine	Dexamethasone	Levomepromazine	177
Diamorphine	Dexamethasone	Metoclopramide	178
Diamorphine	Dexamethasone	Midazolam	179
Diamorphine	Dexamethasone	Ondansetron	179

Drug A	B	C	Page
Diamorphine	Glycopyrronium	Levomepromazine	180
Diamorphine	Glycopyrronium	Midazolam	180
Diamorphine	Glycopyrronium	Ondansetron	181
Diamorphine	Haloperidol	Hyoscine Butylbromide	181
Diamorphine	Haloperidol	Levomepromazine	182
Diamorphine	Haloperidol	Metoclopramide	182
Diamorphine	Haloperidol	Midazolam	183
Diamorphine	Hyoscine Butylbromide	Levomepromazine	184
Diamorphine	Hyoscine Hydrobromide	Levomepromazine	185
Diamorphine	Hyoscine Hydrobromide	Midazolam	186
Diamorphine	Levomepromazine	Metoclopramide	187
Diamorphine	Levomepromazine	Midazolam	188
Diamorphine	Levomepromazine	Octreotide	189
Diamorphine	Metoclopramide	Midazolam	190
Diamorphine	Midazolam	Octreotide	190
Diamorphine	Octreotide	Ranitidine	191
Dihydrocodeine	Cyclizine	Midazolam	191
Dihydrocodeine	Glycopyrronium	Midazolam	191
Fentanyl	Cyclizine	Midazolam	192
Hydromorphone	Cyclizine	Octreotide	192
Hydromorphone	Haloperidol	Hyoscine Hydrobromide	192
Hydromorphone	Hyoscine Hydrobromide	Octreotide	193
Hydromorphone	Ketamine	Midazolam	193
Hydromorphone	Metoclopramide	Midazolam	193
Hydromorphone	Metoclopramide	Ondansetron	194
Methadone	Dexamethasone	Midazolam	194
Methadone	Glycopyrronium	Midazolam	195
Morphine Hydrochloride	Dexamethasone	Haloperidol	195
Morphine Hydrochloride	Dexamethasone	Hyoscine Butylbromide	196
Morphine Hydrochloride	Dexamethasone	Metoclopramide	196
Morphine Hydrochloride	Dexamethasone	Midazolam	197
Morphine Hydrochloride	Haloperidol	Hyoscine Butylbromide	197
Morphine Hydrochloride	Haloperidol	Metoclopramide	198
Morphine Hydrochloride	Haloperidol	Midazolam	198

Drug A	B	C	Page
Morphine Hydrochloride	Hyoscine Butylbromide	Metoclopramide	199
Morphine Hydrochloride	Hyoscine Butylbromide	Midazolam	199
Morphine Hydrochloride	Metoclopramide	Midazolam	199
Morphine Sulphate	Dexamethasone	Haloperidol	200
Morphine Sulphate	Dexamethasone	Metoclopramide	200
Morphine Sulphate	Haloperidol	Hyoscine Hydrobromide	201
Morphine Sulphate	Haloperidol	Ketamine	201
Morphine Sulphate	Haloperidol	Metoclopramide	201
Morphine Sulphate	Hyoscine Butylbromide	Midazolam	202
Morphine Sulphate	Hyoscine Hydrobromide	Midazolam	202
Morphine Sulphate	Hyoscine Hydrobromide	Octreotide	202
Morphine Sulphate	Metoclopramide	Midazolam	203
Morphine Sulphate	Metoclopramide	Ondansetron	204
Morphine Tartrate	Clonazepam	Dexamethasone	204
Morphine Tartrate	Clonazepam	Haloperidol	204
Morphine Tartrate	Clonazepam	Ketamine	205
Morphine Tartrate	Cyclizine	Dexamethasone	205
Morphine Tartrate	Cyclizine	Hyoscine Hydrobromide	206
Morphine Tartrate	Hyoscine Hydrobromide	Midazolam	206
Oxycodone	Clonazepam	Haloperidol	206
Oxycodone	Clonazepam	Hyoscine Butylbromide	207
Oxycodone	Clonazepam	Hyoscine Hydrobromide	207
Oxycodone	Clonazepam	Metoclopramide	208
Oxycodone	Cyclizine	Haloperidol	208
Oxycodone	Haloperidol	Hyoscine Butylbromide	208
Oxycodone	Haloperidol	Hyoscine Hydrobromide	209
Oxycodone	Haloperidol	Ketamine	209
Oxycodone	Haloperidol	Midazolam	209
Oxycodone	Hyoscine Butylbromide	Levomepromazine	210
Oxycodone	Hyoscine Hydrobromide	Levomepromazine	210
Oxycodone	Ketorolac	Ranitidine	211
Oxycodone	Levomepromazine	Octreotide	211
Oxycodone	Octreotide	Ondansetron	211

Drug A	B	C	Page
Tramadol	Dexamethasone	Haloperidol	212
Tramadol	Dexamethasone	Hyoscine Butylbromide	212
Tramadol	Dexamethasone	Metoclopramide	213
Tramadol	Dexamethasone	Midazolam	213
Tramadol	Haloperidol	Hyoscine Butylbromide	214
Tramadol	Haloperidol	Metoclopramide	214
Tramadol	Haloperidol	Midazolam	214
Tramadol	Hyoscine Butylbromide	Metoclopramide	215
Tramadol	Hyoscine Butylbromide	Midazolam	215
Tramadol	Metoclopramide	Midazolam	215
Clonazepam	Haloperidol	Metoclopramide	216
Clonazepam	Hyoscine Hydrobromide	Metoclopramide	216
Cyclizine	Dexamethasone	Hyoscine Butylbromide	217
Cyclizine	Haloperidol	Midazolam	217
Dexamethasone	Haloperidol	Hyoscine Butylbromide	218
Dexamethasone	Haloperidol	Metoclopramide	218
Dexamethasone	Haloperidol	Midazolam	219
Dexamethasone	Hyoscine Butylbromide	Metoclopramide	220
Dexamethasone	Hyoscine Butylbromide	Midazolam	221
Dexamethasone	Metoclopramide	Midazolam	222
Glycopyrronium	Levomepromazine	Octreotide	222
Haloperidol	Hyoscine Butylbromide	Midazolam	223
Hyoscine Butylbromide	Levomepromazine	Octreotide	223
Hyoscine Butylbromide	Metoclopramide	Midazolam	224
Hyoscine Hydrobromide	Ketorolac	Ranitidine	224
Hyoscine Hydrobromide	Levomepromazine	Midazolam	224
Levomepromazine	Metoclopramide	Octreotide	225
Levomepromazine	Midazolam	Octreotide	225
Levomepromazine	Octreotide	Ondansetron	226

Alfentanil (A), Clonazepam (B), and Cyclizine (C)

Summary: No problems with physical stability encountered. Crystallization may occur as concentrations increase. Loss of clonazepam observed when infused via PVC tubing.[1] Minimize loss by using non-PVC tubing.

Drug	Dose in syringe (mg)	Volume in syringe (ml)	Concentration (mg/ml)	Diluent	Outcome	Data Type
A	5		0.29		✓(P) (24 h)	CLIN
B	6	17	0.35	WFI		
C	150		8.82			
A	9		0.53		✓(P) (24 h)	CLIN
B	4	17	0.24	WFI		
C	150		8.82			

Alfentanil (A), Clonazepam (B), and Glycopyrronium (C)

Summary: No problems with physical stability encountered. Loss of clonazepam observed when infused via PVC tubing.[1] Minimize loss by using non-PVC tubing.

Drug	Dose in syringe (mg)	Volume in syringe (ml)	Concentration (mg/ml)	Diluent	Outcome	Data Type
A	10		0.67		✓(P) (24 h)	CLIN
B	4	15	0.27	–		
C	1.8		0.12			
A	12		0.71		✓(P) (24 h)	CLIN
B	4	17	0.24	WFI		
C	0.6		0.04			

Alfentanil (A), Clonazepam (B), and Haloperidol (C)

Summary: No problems with physical stability encountered. Loss of clonazepam observed when infused via PVC tubing.[1] Minimize loss by using non-PVC tubing.

Drug	Dose in syringe (mg)	Volume in syringe (ml)	Concentration (mg/ml)	Diluent	Outcome	Data Type
A	2		0.13		✓ (P)	
B	4	16	0.25	WFI	(24 h)	CLIN
C	5		0.31			
A	6		0.35		✓ (P)	
B	4	17	0.24	NaCl	(24 h)	CLIN
C	10		0.59			

Alfentanil (A), Clonazepam (B), and Hyoscine Hydrobromide (C)

Summary: No problems with physical stability encountered. Loss of clonazepam observed when infused via PVC tubing.[1] Minimize loss by using non-PVC tubing.

Drug	Dose in syringe (mg)	Volume in syringe (ml)	Concentration (mg/ml)	Diluent	Outcome	Data Type
A	2		0.12		✓ (P)	
B	2	17	0.12	WFI	(24 h)	CLIN
C	1.2		0.07			
A	7		0.41		✓ (P)	
B	6	17	0.35	NaCl	(24 h)	CLIN
C	2.4		0.14			
A	10		0.67		✓ (P)	
B	2	15	0.13	WFI	(24 h)	CLIN
C	1.8		0.12			

Alfentanil (A), Cyclizine (B), and Midazolam (C)

Summary: No problems with physical stability encountered. Crystallization may occur as concentrations increase.

Drug	Dose in syringe (mg)	Volume in syringe (ml)	Concentration (mg/ml)	Diluent	Outcome	Data Type
A	3		0.18		✓(P) (24 h)	CLIN
B	150	17	8.82	WFI		
C	20		1.18			
A	55		3.06		✓(P) (24 h)	CLIN
B	75	18	4.17	WFI		
C	20		1.11			
A	75		3.00		✓(P) (24 h)	CLIN
B	150	25	6.00	WFI		
C	30		1.20			

Alfentanil (A), Haloperidol (B), and Midazolam (C)

Summary: No problems with physical stability encountered

Drug	Dose in syringe (mg)	Volume in syringe (ml)	Concentration (mg/ml)	Diluent	Outcome	Data Type
A	5.5		0.32		✓(P) (24 h)	CLIN
B	5	17	0.29	NaCl		
C	40		2.35			
A	14.5		1.12		✓(P) (24 h)	CLIN
B	5	13	0.38	WFI		
C	30		2.31			

Alfentanil (A), Hyoscine Butylbromide (B), and Levomepromazine (C)

Summary: No problems with physical stability encountered. To avoid irritation at the site of infusion, levomepromazine may be given as a subcutaneous bolus injection at doses below 50 mg (= 2 ml).

Drug	Dose in syringe (mg)	Volume in syringe (ml)	Concentration (mg/ml)	Diluent	Outcome	Data Type
A	2.5		0.15		✓ (P)	
B	60	17	3.53	NaCl	(24 h)	CLIN
C	37.5		2.21			
A	6		0.40		✓ (P)	
B	100	15	6.67	WFI	(24 h)	CLIN
C	12.5		0.83			
A	12		0.71		✓ (P)	
B	120	17	7.06	NaCl	(24 h)	CLIN
C	25		1.47			

Alfentanil (A), Levomepromazine (B), and Midazolam (C)

Summary: No problems with physical stability encountered

Drug	Dose in syringe (mg)	Volume in syringe (ml)	Concentration (mg/ml)	Diluent	Outcome	Data Type
A	20		1.67		✓ (P)	
B	50	12	4.17	WFI	(12 h)	CLIN
C	25		2.08			
A	40		1.90		✓ (P)	
B	100	21	4.76	WFI	(24 h)	CLIN
C	40		1.90			
A	8		0.57		✓ (P)	
B	50	14	3.57	NaCl	(24 h)	CLIN
C	25		1.79			

Alfentanil (A), Levomepromazine (B), and Octreotide (C)

Summary: No problems with physical stability encountered

Drug	Dose in syringe (mg)	Volume in syringe (ml)	Concentration (mg/ml)	Diluent	Outcome	Data Type
A	25		1.25			
B	12.5	20	0.63	NaCl	✓ (P) (24 h)	CLIN
C	0.6		0.03			
A	25		1.25			
B	12.5	20	0.63	NaCl	✓ (P) (24 h)	CLIN
C	1		0.05			

Alfentanil (A), Metoclopramide (B), and Midazolam (C)

Summary: No problems with physical stability encountered.

Drug	Dose in syringe (mg)	Volume in syringe (ml)	Concentration (mg/ml)	Diluent	Outcome	Data Type
A	3		0.19			
B	30	16	1.88	WFI	✓ (P) (24 h)	CLIN
C	40		2.50			
A	6		0.35			
B	60	17	3.53	–	✓ (P) (24 h)	CLIN
C	10		0.59			
A	14		1.00			
B	30	14	2.14	WFI	✓ (P) (24 h)	CLIN
C	20		1.43			

Diamorphine (A), Clonazepam (B), and Cyclizine (C)

Summary: No problems with physical stability encountered. Crystallization may occur as concentrations increase. Loss of clonazepam observed when infused via PVC tubing.[1] Minimize loss by using non-PVC tubing.

Drug	Dose in syringe (mg)	Volume in syringe (ml)	Concentration (mg/ml)	Diluent	Outcome	Data Type
A	100		6.67		✓ (P)	
B	4	15	0.27	WFI	(24 h)	CLIN
C	150		10.00			
A	520		30.59		✓ (P)	
B	6	17	0.35	WFI	(24 h)	CLIN
C	150		8.82			

Diamorphine (A), Clonazepam (B), and Dexamethasone (C)

Summary: No problems with physical stability encountered. Dexamethasone is usually given as a subcutaneous bolus injection (depending upon volume of injection) or via a separate CSCI. However, if dexamethasone is to be mixed with other drugs, it should be the last constituent added to the maximally diluted syringe. There may be initial transient turbidity upon the addition of dexamethasone. Loss of clonazepam observed when infused via PVC tubing.[1] Minimize loss by using non-PVC tubing.

Drug	Dose in syringe (mg)	Volume in syringe (ml)	Concentration (mg/ml)	Diluent	Outcome	Data Type
A	20		1.18		✓ (P)	
B	4	17	0.24	WFI	(24 h)	CLIN
C	8		0.47			
A	50		2.94		✓ (P)	
B	2	17	0.12	NaCl	(24 h)	CLIN
C	6		0.35			

Diamorphine (A), Clonazepam (B), and Glycopyrronium (C)

Summary: No problems with physical stability encountered. Loss of clonazepam observed when infused via PVC tubing.[1] Minimize loss by using non-PVC tubing.

Drug	Dose in syringe (mg)	Volume in syringe (ml)	Concentration (mg/ml)	Diluent	Outcome	Data Type
A	10		0.56		✓ (P) (24 h)	
B	5	18	0.28	WFI		CLIN
C	1.2		0.07			
A	60		3.53		✓ (P) (24 h)	
B	2	17	0.12	WFI		CLIN
C	0.6		0.04			

Diamorphine (A), Clonazepam (B), and Haloperidol (C)

Summary: No problems with physical stability encountered. Loss of clonazepam observed when infused via PVC tubing.[1] Minimize loss by using non-PVC tubing.

Drug	Dose in syringe (mg)	Volume in syringe (ml)	Concentration (mg/ml)	Diluent	Outcome	Data Type
A	30		1.76		✓ (P) (24 h)	
B	8	17	0.47	WFI		CLIN
C	5		0.29			
A	20		2.22		✓ (P) (24 h)	
B	1	9	0.11	WFI		CLIN
C	5		0.56			
A	75		4.41		✓ (P) (24 h)	
B	4	17	0.24	NaCl		CLIN
C	10		0.59			

Diamorphine (A), Clonazepam (B), and Hyoscine Butylbromide (C)

Summary: No problems with physical stability encountered. Loss of clonazepam observed when infused via PVC tubing.[1] Minimize loss by using non-PVC tubing.

Drug	Dose in syringe (mg)	Volume in syringe (ml)	Concentration (mg/ml)	Diluent	Outcome	Data Type
A	1800		112.80		✓ (P) (24 h)	CLIN
B	3	16	0.19	WFI		
C	120		7.50			

Diamorphine (A), Clonazepam (B), and Levomepromazine (C)

Summary: No problems with physical stability encountered. To reduce irritation at the site of infusion, levomepromazine may be given as a subcutaneous bolus injection at doses below 50 mg (= 2 ml). Loss of clonazepam observed when infused via PVC tubing.[1] Minimize loss by using non-PVC tubing.

Drug	Dose in syringe (mg)	Volume in syringe (ml)	Concentration (mg/ml)	Diluent	Outcome	Data Type
A	30		1.76		✓ (P) (24 h)	CLIN
B	4	17	0.24	NaCl		
C	12.5		0.74			
A	600		35.29		✓ (P) (24 h)	CLIN
B	3	17	0.18	WFI		
C	18.75		1.10			
A	950		55.88		✓ (P) (24 h)	CLIN
B	2	17	0.12	WFI		
C	25		1.47			

Diamorphine (A), Cyclizine (B), and Dexamethasone (C)

Summary: No problems with physical stability encountered at concentrations below, although the mixture may exhibit concentration-dependent physical incompatibility Dexamethasone is usually given as a subcutaneous bolus injection (depending upon volume of injection) or via a separate CSCI. However, if dexamethasone is to be mixed with other drugs, it should be the last constituent added to the maximally diluted syringe. There may be initial transient turbidity upon the addition of dexamethasone.

Drug	Dose in syringe (mg)	Volume in syringe (ml)	Concentration (mg/ml)	Diluent	Outcome	Data Type
A	80		4.71		✓ (P)	
B	150	17	8.82	WFI	(24 h)	CLIN
C	6		0.35			
A	100		5.88		✓ (P)	
B	150	17	8.82	WFI	(24 h)	CLIN
C	12		0.71			
A	140		8.24		✓ (P)	
B	150	17	8.82	WFI	(24 h)	CLIN
C	8		0.47			
A	250		16.67		✓ (P)	
B	150	15	10.00	WFI	(24 h)	CLIN
C	6		0.40			

Diamorphine (A), Cyclizine (B), and Haloperidol (C)

Summary: No problems with physical stability encountered. Mixture has been shown to be chemically stable, as shown below.[4] Crystallization may occur as concentrations increase.

Drug	Dose in syringe (mg)	Volume in syringe (ml)	Concentration (mg/ml)	Diluent	Outcome	Data Type
A	15		0.88		✓ (P)	
B	150	17	8.82	WFI	(24 h)	CLIN
C	5		0.29			
A	20		1.18		✓ (P)	
B	150	17	8.82	WFI	(24 h)	CLIN
C	15		0.88			
A	50		2.94		✓ (P)	
B	150	17	8.82	WFI	(24 h)	CLIN
C	5		0.29			
A	60		4.00		✓ (P)	
B	150	15	10.00	WFI	(24 h)	CLIN
C	10		0.67			
A	60		6.00		✓ (P)	
B	150	10	15.00	WFI	(24 h)	CLIN
C	10		1.00			
A	150		9.38		✓ (P)	
B	150	16	9.38	WFI	(24 h)	CLIN
C	10		0.63			
A	−		56.00		✓ (P)	
B	−	−	13.00	−	(24 h)	LAB[4]
C	−		2.1			
A	800		57.14		✓ (P)	
B	150	14	10.71	WFI	(24 h)	CLIN
C	10		0.71			

Diamorphine (A), Cyclizine (B), and Hyoscine Butylbromide (C)

Summary: Cyclizine may crystallize with hyoscine butylbromide and/or diamorphine. Problem can be overcome by diluting maximally and changing the antimuscarinic drug to glycopyrronium.

Drug	Dose in syringe (mg)	Volume in syringe (ml)	Concentration (mg/ml)	Diluent	Outcome	Data Type
A	35		2.19			
B	150	16	9.38	WFI	☒	CLIN
C	80		5.00			
A	160		10.67			
B	150	15	10.00	WFI	☒	CLIN
C	40		2.67			

Diamorphine (A), Cyclizine (B), and Hyoscine Hydrobromide (C)

Summary: No problems with physical stability encountered, although crystallization may occur as concentrations increase.

Drug	Dose in syringe (mg)	Volume in syringe (ml)	Concentration (mg/ml)	Diluent	Outcome	Data Type
A	60		3.53			
B	150	17	8.82	WFI	✓ (P) (24 h)	CLIN
C	1.6		0.09			

Diamorphine (A), Cyclizine (B), and Levomepromazine (C)

Summary: No problems with physical stability encountered, although crystallization can occur as concentrations increase. To avoid irritation at the site of infusion, levomepromazine may be given as a subcutaneous bolus injection at doses below 50 mg (= 2 ml). Note that cyclizine and levomepromazine should not usually be administered together.

Drug	Dose in syringe (mg)	Volume in syringe (ml)	Concentration (mg/ml)	Diluent	Outcome	Data Type
A	180		10.56		✓ (P)	
B	150	17	8.82	WFI	(24 h)	CLIN
C	25		1.47			
A	540		31.76		✓ (P)	
B	150	17	8.82	WFI	(24 h)	CLIN
C	100		5.88			

Diamorphine (A), Cyclizine (B), and Metoclopramide (C)

Summary: Crystallization may occur as doses increase. In theory, this is NOT a sensible combination of anti-emetics, since the pro-kinetic action of metoclopramide may (theoretically) be inhibited by cyclizine. Higher doses of metoclopramide may be required to overcome this. However, use of this combination is acceptable if metoclopramide is used for its central dopamine antagonist properties, although haloperidol is preferable.

Drug	Dose in syringe (mg)	Volume in syringe (ml)	Concentration (mg/ml)	Diluent	Outcome	Data Type
A	25		1.47			
B	150	17	8.82	WFI	☒	CLIN
C	40		2.35			
A	40		2.35			
B	200	17	11.76	WFI	☒	CLIN
C	60		3.53			
A	120		7.06		✓ (P)	
B	75	17	4.41	WFI		CLIN
C	30		1.76		(12 h)	

Diamorphine (A), Cyclizine (B), and Midazolam (C)

Summary: No problems with physical stability encountered, although crystallization may occur as concentrations increase.

Drug	Dose in syringe (mg)	Volume in syringe (ml)	Concentration (mg/ml)	Diluent	Outcome	Data Type
A	35		2.06		✓ (P)	
B	150	17	8.82	WFI	(24 h)	CLIN
C	20		1.18			
A	40		2.35		✓ (P)	
B	150	17	8.82	WFI	(24 h)	CLIN
C	30		1.76			
A	60		3.33		✓ (P)	
B	150	18	8.33	WFI	(24 h)	CLIN
C	30		1.67			
A	70		4.12		✓ (P)	
B	150	17	8.82	WFI	(24 h)	CLIN
C	40		2.35			
A	160		9.41		✓ (P)	
B	150	17	8.82	WFI	(24 h)	CLIN
C	30		1.76			
A	320		20.00		✓ (P)	
B	150	16	9.38	WFI	(24 h)	CLIN
C	30		1.88			
A	630		37.06		✓ (P)	
B	150	17	8.82	WFI	(24 h)	CLIN
C	40		2.35			

Diamorphine (A), Dexamethasone (B), and Haloperidol (C)

Summary: No problems with physical stability encountered at concentrations below, although the mixture may exhibit concentration-dependent physical incompatibility. Dexamethasone should be given via a bolus subcutaneous injection, or separate CSCI. However, if dexamethasone is to be mixed with other drugs, it should be the last constituent added to the maximally diluted syringe.

Drug	Dose in syringe (mg)	Volume in syringe (ml)	Concentration (mg/ml)	Diluent	Outcome	Data Type
A	50		2.94			
B	6	17	0.35	WFI	✓ (P) (24 h)	CLIN
C	5		0.29			
A	60		3.53			
B	16	17	0.94	WFI	✓ (P) (24 h)	CLIN
C	5		0.29			
A	100		5.88			
B	8	17	0.47	WFI	✓ (P) (24 h)	CLIN
C	5		0.29			
A	430		25.29			
B	6	17	0.35	WFI	✓ (P) (24 h)	CLIN
C	10		0.59			

Diamorphine (A), Dexamethasone (B), and Hyoscine Hydrobromide (C)

Summary: No problems with physical stability encountered. Dexamethasone is usually given as a subcutaneous bolus injection (depending upon volume of injection) or via a separate CSCI. However, if dexamethasone is to be mixed with other drugs, it should be the last constituent added to the maximally diluted syringe. There may be initial transient turbidity upon the addition of dexamethasone.

Drug	Dose in syringe (mg)	Volume in syringe (ml)	Concentration (mg/ml)	Diluent	Outcome	Data Type
A	20		1.33		✓ (P)	
B	4	15	0.27	WFI	(24 h)	CLIN
C	1.2		0.08			
A	20		1.33		✓ (P)	
B	8	15	0.53	WFI	(24 h)	CLIN
C	0.8		0.05			

Diamorphine (A), Dexamethasone (B), and Levomepromazine (C)

Summary: Physically incompatible at the concentrations listed below. Dexamethasone is usually given as a subcutaneous bolus injection (depending upon volume of injection) or via a separate CSCI. However, if dexamethasone is to be mixed with other drugs, it should be the last constituent added to the maximally diluted syringe. There may be initial transient turbidity upon the addition of dexamethasone. In order to avoid site irritation, levomepromazine may be given as a subcutaneous bolus injection at doses below 50 mg (= 2 ml).

Drug	Dose in syringe (mg)	Volume in syringe (ml)	Concentration (mg/ml)	Diluent	Outcome	Data Type
A	10		0.50			
B	8	20	0.40	WFI	✗	CLIN
C	12.5		0.63			
A	120		7.06			
B	10	17	0.59	WFI	✗	CLIN
C	50		2.94			

Diamorphine (A), Dexamethasone (B), and Metoclopramide (C)

Summary: No problems with physical stability encountered at concentrations below, although the mixture may exhibit concentration-dependent physical incompatibility. Dexamethasone is usually given as a subcutaneous bolus injection (depending upon volume of injection) or via a separate CSCI. However, if dexamethasone is to be mixed with other drugs, it should be the last constituent added to the maximally diluted syringe. There may be initial transient turbidity upon the addition of dexamethasone.

Drug	Dose in syringe (mg)	Volume in syringe (ml)	Concentration (mg/ml)	Diluent	Outcome	Data Type
A	30		1.76		✓ (P) (24 h)	
B	12	17	0.71	WFI		CLIN
C	60		3.53			
A	60		3.53		✓ (P) (24 h)	
B	10	17	0.59	WFI		CLIN
C	40		2.35			
A	150		8.82		✓ (P) (24 h)	
B	4	17	0.24	WFI		CLIN
C	30		1.76			
A	100		5.88		✓ (P) (24 h)	
B	4	17	0.24	WFI		CLIN
C	50		2.94			

Diamorphine (A), Dexamethasone (B), and Midazolam (C)

Summary: No problems with physical stability encountered at concentrations below, although the mixture may exhibit concentration-dependent physical incompatibility. Dexamethasone is usually given as a subcutaneous bolus injection (depending upon volume of injection) or via a separate CSCI. However, if dexamethasone is to be mixed with other drugs, it should be the last constituent added to the maximally diluted syringe. There may be initial transient turbidity upon the addition of dexamethasone. Note that laboratory evidence suggests the possibility of loss of midazolam at a higher temperature (37° C) which may be significant in combinations of midazolam and dexamethasone.[14]

Drug	Dose in syringe (mg)	Volume in syringe (ml)	Concentration (mg/ml)	Diluent	Outcome	Data Type
A	50		2.94		✓ (P)	
B	4	17	0.24	WFI	(24 h)	CLIN
C	20		1.18			

Diamorphine (A), Dexamethasone (B), and Ondansetron (C)

Summary: No problems with physical stability encountered at concentrations below, although the mixture may exhibit concentration-dependent physical incompatibility. Dexamethasone is usually given as a subcutaneous bolus injection (depending upon volume of injection) or via a separate CSCI. However, if dexamethasone is to be mixed with other drugs, it should be the last constituent added to the maximally diluted syringe. There may be initial transient turbidity upon the addition of dexamethasone.

Drug	Dose in syringe (mg)	Volume in syringe (ml)	Concentration (mg/ml)	Diluent	Outcome	Data Type
A	600		35.29		✓ (P)	
B	1	17	0.06	WFI	(24 h)	CLIN
C	24		1.41			

Diamorphine (A), Glycopyrronium (B), and Levomepromazine (C)

Summary: No problems with physical stability encountered. To avoid irritation at the site of infusion, levomepromazine may be given as a subcutaneous bolus injection at doses below 50 mg (= 2 ml).

Drug	Dose in syringe (mg)	Volume in syringe (ml)	Concentration (mg/ml)	Diluent	Outcome	Data Type
A	25		1.56		✓ (P) (24 h)	CLIN
B	0.8	16	0.05	NaCl		
C	25		1.56			
A	30		1.76		✓ (P) (24 h)	CLIN
B	0.8	17	0.05	WFI		
C	12.5		0.74			
A	70		4.12		✓ (P) (24 h)	CLIN
B	1.6	17	0.09	WFI		
C	100		5.88			

Diamorphine (A), Glycopyrronium (B), and Midazolam (C)

Summary: No problems with physical stability encountered.

Drug	Dose in syringe (mg)	Volume in syringe (ml)	Concentration (mg/ml)	Diluent	Outcome	Data Type
A	120		6.67		✓ (P) (24 h)	CLIN
B	1.6	17	0.08	WFI		
C	30		1.33			
A	150		7.89		✓ (P) (24 h)	CLIN
B	2.4	19	0.13	NaCl		
C	20		1.05			
A	420		24.71		✓ (P) (12 h)	CLIN
B	0.8	17	0.05	WFI		
C	40		2.35			

Diamorphine (A), Glycopyrronium (B), and Ondansetron (C)

Summary: No problems with physical stability encountered.

Drug	Dose in syringe (mg)	Volume in syringe (ml)	Concentration (mg/ml)	Diluent	Outcome	Data Type
A	25		1.19		✓ (P)	
B	0.8	21	0.04	NaCl	(24 h)	CLIN
C	24		1.14			
A	75		4.17		✓ (P)	
B	0.6	18	0.03	NaCl	(24 h)	CLIN
C	16		0.89			
A	120		5.71		✓ (P)	
B	1.6	21	0.08	NaCl	(24 h)	CLIN
C	12		0.57			

Diamorphine (A), Haloperidol (B), and Hyoscine Butylbromide (C)

Summary: No problems with physical stability encountered.

Drug	Dose in syringe (mg)	Volume in syringe (ml)	Concentration (mg/ml)	Diluent	Outcome	Data Type
A	30		1.76		✓ (P)	
B	10	17	0.59	WFI	(24 h)	CLIN
C	120		7.06			
A	60		3.53		✓ (P)	
B	10	17	0.59	WFI	(24 h)	CLIN
C	80		4.71			
A	85		5.00		✓ (P)	
B	10	17	0.59	NaCl	(24 h)	CLIN
C	120		7.06			
A	180		10.59		✓ (P)	
B	5	17	0.29	WFI	(24 h)	CLIN
C	80		4.71			

Diamorphine (A), Haloperidol (B), and Levomepromazine (C)

Summary: Although no problems with physical stability were encountered, the use of this combination is not generally recommended because of the increased risk of undesirable effects. To avoid site irritation, levomepromazine can be administered as a subcutaneous bolus injection at doses below 50 mg (= 2 ml).

Drug	Dose in syringe (mg)	Volume in syringe (ml)	Concentration (mg/ml)	Diluent	Outcome	Data Type
A	720		42.35			
B	10	17	0.59	WFI	✓ (P) (24 h)	CLIN
C	200		11.76			

Diamorphine (A), Haloperidol (B), and Metoclopramide (C)

Summary: Although no problems with physical stability were encountered, the use of this combination is not generally recommended because of the increased risk of undesirable effects.

Drug	Dose in syringe (mg)	Volume in syringe (ml)	Concentration (mg/ml)	Diluent	Outcome	Data Type
A	10		0.71			
B	5	14	0.36	WFI	✓ (P) (24 h)	CLIN
C	60		4.29			
A	40		2.35			
B	5	17	0.29	WFI	✓ (P) (24 h)	CLIN
C	30		1.76			
A	80		4.71			
B	10	17	0.59	WFI	✓ (P) (24 h)	CLIN
C	60		3.53			
A	130		7.65			
B	5	17	0.29	WFI	✓ (P) (24 h)	CLIN
C	60		3.53			

Diamorphine (A), Haloperidol (B), and Midazolam (C)

Summary: No problems with physical stability encountered.

Drug	Dose in syringe (mg)	Volume in syringe (ml)	Concentration (mg/ml)	Diluent	Outcome	Data Type
A	20		1.18		✔ (P)	
B	5	17	0.29	WFI	(24 h)	CLIN
C	30		1.76			
A	40		2.35		✔ (P)	
B	2.5	17	0.15	WFI	(24 h)	CLIN
C	20		1.18			
A	120		7.06		✔ (P)	
B	5	17	0.29	WFI	(24 h)	CLIN
C	30		1.76			
A	450		26.47		✔ (P)	
B	5	17	0.29	WFI	(24 h)	CLIN
C	20		1.18			
A	630		37.06		✔ (P)	
B	10	17	0.59	WFI	(24 h)	CLIN
C	30		1.76			
A	840		49.41		✔ (P)	
B	10	17	0.59	WFI	(24 h)	CLIN
C	40		2.35			

Diamorphine (A), Hyoscine Butylbromide (B), and Levomepromazine (C)

Summary: No problems with physical stability encountered. To avoid irritation at the site of infusion, levomepromazine may be given as a subcutaneous bolus injection at doses below 50 mg (= 2 ml).

Drug	Dose in syringe (mg)	Volume in syringe (ml)	Concentration (mg/ml)	Diluent	Outcome	Data Type
A	40		2.35		✓ (P) (24 h)	CLIN
B	120	17	7.06	WFI		
C	6.25		0.37			
A	45		2.81		✓ (P) (24 h)	CLIN
B	120	16	7.50	NaCl		
C	12.5		0.78			
A	100		5.88		✓ (P) (24 h)	CLIN
B	80	17	4.71	WFI		
C	25		1.47			
A	120		7.06		✓ (P) (24 h)	CLIN
B	120	17	7.06	WFI		
C	50		2.94			
A	350		20.59		✓ (P) (24 h)	CLIN
B	80	17	4.71	WFI		
C	50		2.94			
A	1400		82.35		✓ (P) (24 h)	CLIN
B	120	17	7.06	WFI		
C	37.50		2.21			
A	1900		111.76		✓ (P) (24 h)	CLIN
B	120	17	7.06	WFI		
C	50		2.94			

Diamorphine (A), Hyoscine Hydrobromide (B), and Levomepromazine (C)

Summary: No problems with physical stability encountered. To avoid irritation at the site of infusion, levomepromazine may be given as a subcutaneous bolus injection at doses below 50 mg (= 2 ml).

Drug	Dose in syringe (mg)	Volume in syringe (ml)	Concentration (mg/ml)	Diluent	Outcome	Data Type
A	15		0.88		✓ (P)	
B	0.8	17	0.05	NaCl	(24 h)	CLIN
C	25		1.47			
A	80		4.71		✓ (P)	
B	1.8	17	0.11	WFI	(24 h)	CLIN
C	75		4.41			
A	450		26.47		✓ (P)	
B	2.4	17	0.14	WFI	(24 h)	CLIN
C	100		5.88			

Diamorphine (A), Hyoscine Hydrobromide (B), and Midazolam (C)

Summary: No problems with physical stability encountered.

Drug	Dose in syringe (mg)	Volume in syringe (ml)	Concentration (mg/ml)	Diluent	Outcome	Data Type
A	50		2.94		✓ (P) (24 h)	
B	2.4	17	0.14	WFI		CLIN
C	20		1.18			
A	70		4.12		✓ (P) (24 h)	
B	1.2	17	0.07	WFI		CLIN
C	30		1.76			
A	80		4.71		✓ (P) (24 h)	
B	1.6	17	0.09	WFI		CLIN
C	20		1.18			
A	160		9.41		✓ (P) (24 h)	
B	1.2	17	0.07	WFI		CLIN
C	30		1.76			
A	200		11.76		✓ (P) (24 h)	
B	1.2	17	0.07	WFI		CLIN
C	30		1.76			
A	420		24.71		✓ (P) (24 h)	
B	1.6	17	0.09	WFI		CLIN
C	40		2.35			
A	720		42.35		✓ (P) (24 h)	
B	1.6	17	0.09	WFI		CLIN
C	40		2.35			

Diamorphine (A), Levomepromazine (B), and Metoclopramide (C)

Summary: No problems with physical stability encountered. To avoid irritation at the site of infusion, levomepromazine may be given as a subcutaneous bolus injection at doses below 50 mg (= 2 ml). Note that levomepromazine can antagonize the prokinetic effect of metoclopramide and this combination may lead to an increased risk of undesirable effects.

Drug	Dose in syringe (mg)	Volume in syringe (ml)	Concentration (mg/ml)	Diluent	Outcome	Data Type
A	50		2.94		✓ (P)	
B	75	17	4.41	WFI	(24 h)	CLIN
C	60		3.53			
A	70		4.12		✓ (P)	
B	12.5	17	0.74	WFI	(24 h)	CLIN
C	40		2.35			
A	100		5.88		✓ (P)	
B	25	17	1.47	NaCl	(24 h)	CLIN
C	30		1.76			
A	250		14.71		✓ (P)	
B	50	17	2.94	WFI	(24 h)	CLIN
C	60		3.53			

Diamorphine (A), Levomepromazine (B), and Midazolam (C)

Summary: No problems with physical stability encountered. To avoid irritation at the site of infusion, levomepromazine may be given as a subcutaneous bolus injection at doses below 50 mg (= 2ml).

Drug	Dose in syringe (mg)	Volume in syringe (ml)	Concentration (mg/ml)	Diluent	Outcome	Data Type
A	60		3.53		✓ (P) (24 h)	
B	125	17	7.35	WFI		CLIN
C	25		1.47			
A	1450		85.29		✓ (P) (24 h)	
B	12.5	17	0.74	WFI		CLIN
C	30		1.76			
A	1600		94.12		✓ (P) (24 h)	
B	50	17	2.94	WFI		CLIN
C	30		1.76			
A	2400		137.14		✓ (P) (24 h)	
B	60	17.5	3.43	WFI		CLIN
C	37.5		2.14			

Diamorphine (A), Levomepromazine (B), and Octreotide (C)

Summary: No problems with physical stability encountered. To avoid irritation at the site of infusion, levomepromazine may be given as a subcutaneous bolus injection at doses below 50 mg (= 2 ml).

Drug	Dose in syringe (mg)	Volume in syringe (ml)	Concentration (mg/ml)	Diluent	Outcome	Data Type
A	50		2.94		✓ (P)	
B	37.5	17	2.41	WFI	(24 h)	CLIN
C	0.60		0.04			
A	80		4.71		✓ (P)	
B	50	17	2.94	WFI	(24 h)	CLIN
C	0.60		0.04			
A	130		7.65		✓ (P)	
B	12.5	17	0.74	NaCl	(24 h)	CLIN
C	0.6		0.04			
A	170		10.00		✓ (P)	
B	75	17	4.41	WFI	(24 h)	CLIN
C	1.00		0.06			

Diamorphine (A), Metoclopramide (B), and Midazolam (C)

Summary: No problems with physical stability encountered.

Drug	Dose in syringe (mg)	Volume in syringe (ml)	Concentration (mg/ml)	Diluent	Outcome	Data Type
A	50		2.94		✓ (P) (24 h)	CLIN
B	30	17	1.76	WFI		
C	10		0.59			
A	180		10.59		✓ (P) (24 h)	CLIN
B	20	17	1.18	WFI		
C	40		2.35			
A	250		14.71		✓ (P) (24 h)	CLIN
B	40	17	2.35	WFI		
C	30		1.76			
A	420		24.71		✓ (P) (24 h)	CLIN
B	60	17	3.53	WFI		
C	20		1.18			

Diamorphine (A), Midazolam (B), and Octreotide (C)

Summary: No problems with physical stability encountered.

Drug	Dose in syringe (mg)	Volume in syringe (ml)	Concentration (mg/ml)	Diluent	Outcome	Data Type
A	75		4.41		✓ (P) (24 h)	CLIN
B	20	17	1.18	NaCl		
C	0.3		0.02			
A	140		8.24		✓ (P) (24 h)	CLIN
B	40	17	2.35	WFI		
C	0.6		0.04			

Diamorphine (A), Octreotide (B), and Ranitidine (C)

Summary: No problems with physical stability encountered.

Drug	Dose in syringe (mg)	Volume in syringe (ml)	Concentration (mg/ml)	Diluent	Outcome	Data Type
A	20		1.05		✓ (P)	
B	0.6	19	0.03	NaCl	(24 h)	CLIN
C	150		7.89			
A	70		4.12		✓ (P)	
B	0.6	17	0.04	NaCl	(24 h)	CLIN
C	150		8.82			

Dihydrocodeine (A), Cyclizine (B), and Midazolam (C)

Summary: No problems with physical stability encountered.

Drug	Dose in syringe (mg)	Volume in syringe (ml)	Concentration (mg/ml)	Diluent	Outcome	Data Type
A	100		7.14		✓ (P)	
B	150	14	10.71	WFI	(24 h)	CLIN
C	10		0.71			

Dihydrocodeine (A), Glycopyrronium (B), and Midazolam (C)

Summary: No problems with physical stability encountered.

Drug	Dose in syringe (mg)	Volume in syringe (ml)	Concentration (mg/ml)	Diluent	Outcome	Data Type
A	50		5.00		✓ (P)	
B	0.8	10	0.08	WFI	(24 h)	CLIN
C	20		2.00			

Fentanyl (A), Cyclizine (B), and Midazolam (C)

Summary: No problems with physical stability encountered.

Drug	Dose in syringe (mg)	Volume in syringe (ml)	Concentration (mg/ml)	Diluent	Outcome	Data Type
A	0.6		0.03			
B	100	18	5.56	WFI	✓ (P) (24 h)	CLIN
C	2.5		0.14			

Hydromorphone (A), Cyclizine (B), and Octreotide (C)

Summary: No problems with physical stability encountered.

Drug	Dose in syringe (mg)	Volume in syringe (ml)	Concentration (mg/ml)	Diluent	Outcome	Data Type
A	30		1.67			
B	300	18	16.67	WFI	✓ (P) (24 h)	CLIN
C	0.40		0.02			

Hydromorphone (A), Haloperidol (B), and Hyoscine Hydrobromide (C)

Summary: No problems with physical stability encountered.

Drug	Dose in syringe (mg)	Volume in syringe (ml)	Concentration (mg/ml)	Diluent	Outcome	Data Type
A	100		14.29			
B	10	7	1.43	DEX	✓ (P) (24 h)	LAB
C	1.2		0.17			

Hydromorphone (A), Hyoscine Hydrobromide (B), and Octreotide (C)

Summary: No problems with physical stability encountered.

Drug	Dose in syringe (mg)	Volume in syringe (ml)	Concentration (mg/ml)	Diluent	Outcome	Data Type
A	100		18.87		✓ (P)	
B	1.2	5.3	0.23	DEX	(24 h)	LAB
C	0.3		0.06			

Hydromorphone (A), Ketamine (B), and Midazolam (C)

Summary: No problems with physical stability encountered.

Drug	Dose in syringe (mg)	Volume in syringe (ml)	Concentration (mg/ml)	Diluent	Outcome	Data Type
A	28		1.56		✓ (P)	
B	50	18	2.78	NaCl	(24 h)	CLIN
C	5		0.28			
A	28		1.56		✓ (P)	
B	300	18	16.67	NaCl	(24 h)	CLIN
C	5		0.28			
A	120		6.67		✓ (P)	
B	100	18	5.56	–	(24 h)	CLIN
C	20		1.11			

Hydromorphone (A), Metoclopramide (B), and Midazolam (C)

Summary: No problems with physical stability encountered.

Drug	Dose in syringe (mg)	Volume in syringe (ml)	Concentration (mg/ml)	Diluent	Outcome	Data Type
A	6		0.33		✓ (P)	
B	20	18	1.11	NaCl	(24 h)	CLIN
C	2.5		0.14			

Hydromorphone (A), Metoclopramide (B), and Ondansetron (C)

Summary: No problems with physical stability encountered.

Drug	Dose in syringe (mg)	Volume in syringe (ml)	Concentration (mg/ml)	Diluent	Outcome	Data Type
A	200		11.11		✓ (P)	
B	30	18	1.67	DEX	(24 h)	LAB
C	16		0.89			

Methadone (A), Dexamethasone (B), and Midazolam (C)

Summary: No problems with physical stability encountered at concentrations below, although the mixture may exhibit concentration-dependent physical incompatibility. Dexamethasone is usually given as a subcutaneous bolus injection (depending upon volume of injection) or via a separate CSCI. However, if dexamethasone is to be mixed with other drugs, it should be the last constituent added to the maximally diluted syringe. There may be initial transient turbidity upon the addition of dexamethasone. Note that laboratory evidence suggests the possibility of loss of midazolam at a higher temperature (37° C) which may be significant in combinations of midazolam and dexamethasone.[14]

Drug	Dose in syringe (mg)	Volume in syringe (ml)	Concentration (mg/ml)	Diluent	Outcome	Data Type
A	4		0.24		✓ (P)	
B	1	17	0.06	WFI	(24 h)	CLIN
C	20		1.18			

Methadone (A), Glycopyrronium (B), and Midazolam (C)

Summary: No problems with physical stability encountered. Site irritation can be a problem with methadone.

Drug	Dose in syringe (mg)	Volume in syringe (ml)	Concentration (mg/ml)	Diluent	Outcome	Data Type
A	40		2.00		✓ (P)	
B	1.2	20	0.06	NaCl	(24 h)	CLIN
C	40		2.00			
A	50		2.50		✓ (P)	
B	0.8	20	0.04	NaCl	(24 h)	CLIN
C	20		1.00			

Morphine Hydrochloride (A), Dexamethasone (B), and Haloperidol (C)

Summary: Physically incompatible at these concentrations. Dexamethasone is usually given as a subcutaneous bolus injection (depending upon volume of injection) or via a separate CSCI. However, if dexamethasone is to be mixed with other drugs, it should be the last constituent added to the maximally diluted syringe. There may be initial transient turbidity upon the addition of dexamethasone.

Drug	Dose in syringe (mg)	Volume in syringe (ml)	Concentration (mg/ml)	Diluent	Outcome	Data Type
A	300		5.00			
B	80	60	1.33	NaCl	✗[†]	LAB[11]
C	37.5		0.63			

[†]Infusion rate set at 0.5 ml/hour over the 5 days.

Morphine Hydrochloride (A), Dexamethasone (B), and Hyoscine Butylbromide (C)

Summary: No problems with physical stability encountered. Dexamethasone is usually given as a subcutaneous bolus injection (depending upon volume of injection) or via a separate CSCI. However, if dexamethasone is to be mixed with other drugs, it should be the last constituent added to the maximally diluted syringe. There may be initial transient turbidity upon the addition of dexamethasone.

Drug	Dose in syringe (mg)	Volume in syringe (ml)	Concentration (mg/ml)	Diluent	Outcome	Data Type
A	300		5.00		✓ (P)	
B	80	60	1.33	NaCl		LAB[11]
C	300		5.00		(5 days)[†]	

[†]Infusion rate set at 0.5 ml/hour over the 5 days.

Morphine Hydrochloride (A), Dexamethasone (B), and Metoclopramide (C)

Summary: No problems with physical stability encountered at concentrations below, although the mixture may exhibit concentration-dependent physical incompatibility. Dexamethasone is usually given as a subcutaneous bolus injection (depending upon volume of injection) or via a separate CSCI. However, if dexamethasone is to be mixed with other drugs, it should be the last constituent added to the maximally diluted syringe. There may be initial transient turbidity upon the addition of dexamethasone.

Drug	Dose in syringe (mg)	Volume in syringe (ml)	Concentration (mg/ml)	Diluent	Outcome	Data Type
A	420		1.68		✓ (P)	
B	112	250	0.45	NaCl		LAB[11]
C	280		1.12		(7 days)[†]	

[†]Infusion rate set at 1.5 ml/hour over the 7 days.

Morphine Hydrochloride (A), Dexamethasone (B), and Midazolam (C)

Summary: Physically incompatible at these concentrations. Dexamethasone is usually given as a subcutaneous bolus injection (depending upon volume of injection) or via a separate CSCI. However, if dexamethasone is to be mixed with other drugs, it should be the last constituent added to the maximally diluted syringe. There may be initial transient turbidity upon the addition of dexamethasone. Laboratory study suggests possibility of loss of midazolam at higher temperature (37° C) which may be significant in combinations of midazolam and dexamethasone.[14]

Drug	Dose in syringe (mg)	Volume in syringe (ml)	Concentration (mg/ml)	Diluent	Outcome	Data Type
A	300		5.00			
B	80	60	1.33	NaCl	☒[†]	LAB[11]
C	75		1.25			

[†]Infusion rate set at 0.5 ml/hour over the 5 days.

Morphine Hydrochloride (A), Haloperidol (B), and Hyoscine Butylbromide (C)

Summary: No problems with physical stability encountered.

Drug	Dose in syringe (mg)	Volume in syringe (ml)	Concentration (mg/ml)	Diluent	Outcome	Data Type
A	300		5.00		✓ (P)	
B	37.5	60	0.63	NaCl	(5 days)[†]	LAB[11]
C	300		5.00			

[†]Infusion rate set at 0.5 ml/hour over the 5 days.

Morphine Hydrochloride (A), Haloperidol (B), and Metoclopramide (C)

Summary: Although no problems with physical stability were encountered, the use of this combination of anti-emetics is not generally recommended because of the increased risk of undesirable effects.

Drug	Dose in syringe (mg)	Volume in syringe (ml)	Concentration (mg/ml)	Diluent	Outcome	Data Type
A	420		1.68		✓ (P)	
B	52.5	250	0.21	NaCl		LAB[11]
C	280		1.12		(7 days)[†]	

[†]Infusion rate set at 1.5 ml/hour over the 7 days.

Morphine Hydrochloride (A), Haloperidol (B), and Midazolam (C)

Summary: No problems with physical stability encountered.

Drug	Dose in syringe (mg)	Volume in syringe (ml)	Concentration (mg/ml)	Diluent	Outcome	Data Type
A	300		5.00		✓ (P)	
B	37.5	60	0.63	NaCl		LAB[11]
C	75		1.25		(5 days)[†]	

[†]Infusion rate set at 0.5 ml/hour over the 5 days.

Morphine Hydrochloride (A), Hyoscine Butylbromide (B), and Metoclopramide (C)

Summary: No problems with physical stability encountered. This is NOT a sensible combination of anti-emetics, since the pro-kinetic action of metoclopramide is inhibited by hyoscine. Higher doses of metoclopramide will be required to overcome this. However, use of this combination is acceptable if metoclopramide is used for its central dopamine antagonist properties, although haloperidol is the preferred choice.

Drug	Dose in syringe (mg)	Volume in syringe (ml)	Concentration (mg/ml)	Diluent	Outcome	Data Type
A	420		1.68		✓ (P)	
B	420	250	1.68	NaCl	(7 days)†	LAB[11]
C	280		1.12			

†Infusion rate set at 1.5 ml/hour over the 7 days.

Morphine Hydrochloride (A), Hyoscine Butylbromide (B), and Midazolam (C)

Summary: No problems with physical stability encountered.

Drug	Dose in syringe (mg)	Volume in syringe (ml)	Concentration (mg/ml)	Diluent	Outcome	Data Type
A	300		5.00		✓ (P)	
B	300	60	5.00	NaCl	(5 days)†	LAB[11]
C	75		1.25			

†Infusion rate set at 0.5 ml/hour over the 5 days.

Morphine Hydrochloride (A), Metoclopramide (B), and Midazolam (C)

Summary: No problems with physical stability encountered.

Drug	Dose in syringe (mg)	Volume in syringe (ml)	Concentration (mg/ml)	Diluent	Outcome	Data Type
A	420		1.68		✓ (P)	
B	280	250	1.12	NaCl	(7 days)†	LAB[11]
C	105		0.42			

†Infusion rate set at 1.5 ml/hour over the 7 days.

Morphine Sulphate (A), Dexamethasone (B), and Haloperidol (C)

Summary: No problems with physical stability encountered at concentrations below, although the mixture may exhibit concentration-dependent physical incompatibility. Dexamethasone is usually given as a subcutaneous bolus injection (depending upon volume of injection) or via a separate CSCI. However, if dexamethasone is to be mixed with other drugs, it should be the last constituent added to the maximally diluted syringe. There may be initial transient turbidity upon the addition of dexamethasone.

Drug	Dose in syringe (mg)	Volume in syringe (ml)	Concentration (mg/ml)	Diluent	Outcome	Data Type
A	60		3.33			
B	4	18	0.22	NaCl	✓ (P) (24 h)	CLIN
C	4		0.22			

Morphine Sulphate (A), Dexamethasone (B), and Metoclopramide (C)

Summary: No problems with physical stability encountered at concentrations below, although the mixture may exhibit concentration-dependent physical incompatibility. Dexamethasone is usually given as a subcutaneous bolus injection (depending upon volume of injection) or via a separate CSCI. However, if dexamethasone is to be mixed with other drugs, it should be the last constituent added to the maximally diluted syringe. There may be initial transient turbidity upon the addition of dexamethasone.

Drug	Dose in syringe (mg)	Volume in syringe (ml)	Concentration (mg/ml)	Diluent	Outcome	Data Type
A	15		0.83			
B	8	18	0.44	NaCl	✓ (P) (24 h)	CLIN
C	30		1.67			
A	30		1.67			
B	16	18	0.89	NaCl	✓ (P) (24 h)	CLIN
C	60		3.33			

Morphine Tartrate (A), Clonazepam (B), and Ketamine (C)

Summary: No problems with physical stability encountered. Loss of clonazepam observed when infused via PVC tubing.[1] Minimize loss by using non-PVC tubing.

Drug	Dose in syringe (mg)	Volume in syringe (ml)	Concentration (mg/ml)	Diluent	Outcome	Data Type
A	540		30.00		✓ (P)	
B	5	18	0.28	NaCl	(24 h)	CLIN
C	100		5.56			
A	750		41.67		✓ (P)	
B	3	18	0.17	NaCl	(24 h)	CLIN
C	400		22.22			
A	800		44.44		✓ (P)	
B	2	18	0.11	NaCl	(24 h)	CLIN
C	200		11.11			

Morphine Tartrate (A), Cyclizine (B), and Dexamethasone (C)

Summary: No problems with physical stability encountered at concentrations below, although the mixture may exhibit concentration-dependent physical incompatibility. Dexamethasone is usually given as a subcutaneous bolus injection (depending upon volume of injection) or via a separate CSCI. However, if dexamethasone is to be mixed with other drugs, it should be the last constituent added to the maximally diluted syringe. There may be initial transient turbidity upon the addition of dexamethasone.

Drug	Dose in syringe (mg)	Volume in syringe (ml)	Concentration (mg/ml)	Diluent	Outcome	Data Type
A	200		11.11		✓ (P)	
B	100	18	5.56	WFI	(24 h)	CLIN
C	8		0.44			

Morphine Tartrate (A), Cyclizine (B), and Hyoscine Hydrobromide (C)

Summary: No problems with physical stability encountered.

Drug	Dose in syringe (mg)	Volume in syringe (ml)	Concentration (mg/ml)	Diluent	Outcome	Data Type
A	900		50.00		✓ (P)	
B	50	18	2.78	WFI	(24 h)	CLIN
C	0.2		0.01			
A	1100		61.11		✓ (P)	
B	50	18	2.78	WFI	(24 h)	CLIN
C	0.2		0.01			

Morphine Tartrate (A), Hyoscine Hydrobromide (B), and Midazolam (C)

Summary: No problems with physical stability encountered.

Drug	Dose in syringe (mg)	Volume in syringe (ml)	Concentration (mg/ml)	Diluent	Outcome	Data Type
A	150		8.33		✓ (P)	
B	0.6	18	0.03	NaCl	(24 h)	CLIN
C	10		0.56			

Oxycodone (A), Clonazepam (B), and Haloperidol (C)

Summary: No problems with physical stability encountered. Loss of clonazepam observed when infused via PVC tubing.[1] Minimize loss by using non-PVC tubing.

Drug	Dose in syringe (mg)	Volume in syringe (ml)	Concentration (mg/ml)	Diluent	Outcome	Data Type
A	100		5.00		✓ (P)	
B	2	20	0.10	WFI	(24 h)	LAB[12]
C	10		0.50			
A	100		5.00		✓ (P)	
B	2	20	0.10	NaCl	(24 h)	LAB[12]
C	10		0.50			

Oxycodone (A), Clonazepam (B), and Hyoscine Butylbromide (C)

Summary: No problems with physical stability encountered. Loss of clonazepam observed when infused via PVC tubing.[1] Minimize loss by using non-PVC tubing.

Drug	Dose in syringe (mg)	Volume in syringe (ml)	Concentration (mg/ml)	Diluent	Outcome	Data Type
A	100		5.00		✓ (P)	
B	2	20	0.10	WFI	(24 h)	LAB[12]
C	100		5.00			
A	100		5.00		✓ (P)	
B	2	20	0.10	NaCl	(24 h)	LAB[12]
C	100		5.00			

Oxycodone (A), Clonazepam (B), and Hyoscine Hydrobromide (C)

Summary: No problems with physical stability encountered. Loss of clonazepam observed when infused via PVC tubing.[1] Minimize loss by using non-PVC tubing.

Drug	Dose in syringe (mg)	Volume in syringe (ml)	Concentration (mg/ml)	Diluent	Outcome	Data Type
A	100		5.00		✓ (P)	
B	2	20	0.10	WFI	(24 h)	LAB[12]
C	1.2		0.06			
A	100		5.00		✓ (P)	
B	2	20	0.10	NaCl	(24 h)	LAB[12]
C	1.2		0.06			

Oxycodone (A), Clonazepam (B), and Metoclopramide (C)

Summary: No problems with physical stability encountered. Loss of clonazepam observed when infused via PVC tubing.[1] Minimize loss by using non-PVC tubing.

Drug	Dose in syringe (mg)	Volume in syringe (ml)	Concentration (mg/ml)	Diluent	Outcome	Data Type
A	100		5.00			
B	2	20	0.10	WFI	✓(P) (24 h)	LAB[12]
C	20		1.00			
A	100		5.00			
B	2	20	0.10	NaCl	✓(P) (24 h)	LAB[12]
C	20		1.00			

Oxycodone (A), Cyclizine (B), and Haloperidol (C)

Summary: No problems with physical stability encountered. Crystallization may occur as concentrations increase.

Drug	Dose in syringe (mg)	Volume in syringe (ml)	Concentration (mg/ml)	Diluent	Outcome	Data Type
A	25		1.47			
B	150	17	8.82	WFI	✓(P) (24 h)	CLIN
C	5		0.29			

Oxycodone (A), Haloperidol (B), and Hyoscine Butylbromide (C)

Summary: No problems with physical stability encountered.

Drug	Dose in syringe (mg)	Volume in syringe (ml)	Concentration (mg/ml)	Diluent	Outcome	Data Type
A	100		5.00			
B	5	20	0.25	WFI	✓(P) (24 h)	LAB[12]
C	120		6.00			
A	100		5.00			
B	5	20	0.25	NaCl	✓(P) (24 h)	LAB[12]
C	120		6.00			

Oxycodone (A), Haloperidol (B), and Hyoscine Hydrobromide (C)

Summary: No problems with physical stability encountered.

Drug	Dose in syringe (mg)	Volume in syringe (ml)	Concentration (mg/ml)	Diluent	Outcome	Data Type
A	100		5.00		✓ (P)	
B	5	20	0.25	WFI	(24 h)	LAB[12]
C	1.2		0.06			
A	100		5.00		✓ (P)	
B	5	20	0.25	NaCl	(24 h)	LAB[12]
C	1.2		0.06			

Oxycodone (A), Haloperidol (B), and Ketamine (C)

Summary: No problems with physical stability encountered.

Drug	Dose in syringe (mg)	Volume in syringe (ml)	Concentration (mg/ml)	Diluent	Outcome	Data Type
A	100		5.00		✓ (P)	
B	5	20	0.25	WFI	(24 h)	LAB[12]
C	150		7.50			
A	100		5.00		✓ (P)	
B	5	20	0.25	NaCl	(24 h)	LAB[12]
C	150		7.50			

Oxycodone (A), Haloperidol (B), and Midazolam (C)

Summary: No problems with physical stability encountered.

Drug	Dose in syringe (mg)	Volume in syringe (ml)	Concentration (mg/ml)	Diluent	Outcome	Data Type
A	100		5.00		✓ (P)	
B	5	20	0.25	WFI	(24 h)	LAB[12]
C	20		1.00			
A	100		5.00		✓ (P)	
B	5	20	0.25	NaCl	(24 h)	LAB[12]
C	20		1.00			

Oxycodone (A), Hyoscine Butylbromide (B), and Levomepromazine (C) B

Summary: No problems with physical stability encountered. To reduce irritation at the site of infusion, levomepromazine may be given as a subcutaneous bolus injection at doses below 50 mg (= 2 ml).

Drug	Dose in syringe (mg)	Volume in syringe (ml)	Concentration (mg/ml)	Diluent	Outcome	Data Type
A	100		5.00		✓ (P)	
B	25	20	1.25	WFI	(24 h)	LAB[12]
C	120		6.00			
A	100		5.00		✓ (P)	
B	25	20	1.25	NaCl	(24 h)	LAB[12]
C	120		6.00			

Oxycodone (A), Hyoscine Hydrobromide (B), and Levomepromazine (C) B

Summary: No problems with physical stability encountered. To reduce irritation at the site of infusion, levomepromazine may be given as a subcutaneous bolus injection at doses below 50 mg (= 2 ml).

Drug	Dose in syringe (mg)	Volume in syringe (ml)	Concentration (mg/ml)	Diluent	Outcome	Data Type
A	100		5.00		✓ (P)	
B	25	20	1.25	WFI	(24 h)	LAB[12]
C	1.2		0.06			
A	100		5.00		✓ (P)	
B	25	20	1.25	NaCl	(24 h)	LAB[12]
C	1.2		0.06			

Oxycodone (A), Ketorolac (B), and Ranitidine (C)

Summary: No problems with physical stability encountered.

Drug	Dose in syringe (mg)	Volume in syringe (ml)	Concentration (mg/ml)	Diluent	Outcome	Data Type
A	100		5.00		✓ (P)	
B	90	20	4.50	WFI	(24 h)	LAB[12]
C	150		7.50			
A	100		5.00		✓ (P)	
B	90	20	4.50	NaCl	(24 h)	LAB[12]
C	150		7.50			

Oxycodone (A), Levomepromazine (B), and Octreotide (C)

Summary: No problems with physical stability encountered. To avoid irritation at the site of infusion, levomepromazine may be given as a subcutaneous bolus injection at doses below 50 mg (= 2 ml).

Drug	Dose in syringe (mg)	Volume in syringe (ml)	Concentration (mg/ml)	Diluent	Outcome	Data Type
A	100		5.00		✓ (P)	
B	25	20	1.25	WFI	(24 h)	LAB[12]
C	0.5		0.03			
A	100		5.00		✓ (P)	
B	25	20	1.25	NaCl	(24 h)	LAB[12]
C	0.5		0.03			

Oxycodone (A), Octreotide (B), and Ondansetron (C)

Summary: No problems with physical stability encountered.

Drug	Dose in syringe (mg)	Volume in syringe (ml)	Concentration (mg/ml)	Diluent	Outcome	Data Type
A	100		5.00		✓ (P)	
B	0.5	20	0.03	WFI	(24 h)	LAB[12]
C	16		0.80			
A	100		5.00		✓ (P)	
B	0.5	20	0.03	NaCl	(24 h)	LAB[12]
C	16		0.80			

Tramadol (A), Dexamethasone (B), and Haloperidol (C)

Summary: Physically incompatible at these concentrations. Dexamethasone is usually given as a subcutaneous bolus injection (depending upon volume of injection) or via a separate CSCI. However, if dexamethasone is to be mixed with other drugs, it should be the last constituent added to the maximally diluted syringe. There may be initial transient turbidity upon the addition of dexamethasone.

Drug	Dose in syringe (mg)	Volume in syringe (ml)	Concentration (mg/ml)	Diluent	Outcome	Data Type
A	2000		33.33			
B	80	60	1.33	NaCl	✗[†]	LAB[11]
C	37.5		0.63			

[†]Infusion rate set at 0.5 ml/hour over the 5 days.

Tramadol (A), Dexamethasone (B), and Hyoscine Butylbromide (C)

Summary: No problems with physical stability encountered at concentrations below, although the mixture may exhibit concentration-dependent physical incompatibility. Dexamethasone is usually given as a subcutaneous bolus injection (depending upon volume of injection) or via a separate CSCI. However, if dexamethasone is to be mixed with other drugs, it should be the last constituent added to the maximally diluted syringe. There may be initial transient turbidity upon the addition of dexamethasone.

Drug	Dose in syringe (mg)	Volume in syringe (ml)	Concentration (mg/ml)	Diluent	Outcome	Data Type
A	2800		11.20		✓(P)	
B	112	250	0.45	NaCl	(7 days)[†]	LAB[11]
C	420		1.68			

[†]Infusion rate set at 1.5 ml/hour over the 7 days.

Tramadol (A), Dexamethasone (B), and Metoclopramide (C)

Summary: No problems with physical stability encountered at concentrations below, although the mixture may exhibit concentration-dependent physical incompatibility. Dexamethasone is usually given as a subcutaneous bolus injection (depending upon volume of injection) or via a separate CSCI. However, if dexamethasone is to be mixed with other drugs, it should be the last constituent added to the maximally diluted syringe. There may be initial transient turbidity upon the addition of dexamethasone.

Drug	Dose in syringe (mg)	Volume in syringe (ml)	Concentration (mg/ml)	Diluent	Outcome	Data Type
A	2800		11.20		✓ (P)	
B	112	250	0.45	NaCl	(7 days)[†]	LAB[11]
C	280		1.12			

[†]Infusion rate set at 1.5 ml/hour over the 7 days.

Tramadol (A), Dexamethasone (B), and Midazolam (C)

Summary: Physically incompatible at these concentrations. Dexamethasone is usually given as a subcutaneous bolus injection (depending upon volume of injection) or via a separate CSCI. However, if dexamethasone is to be mixed with other drugs, it should be the last constituent added to the maximally diluted syringe. There may be initial transient turbidity upon the addition of dexamethasone. Laboratory study suggests possibility of loss of midazolam at higher temperature (37° C) which may be significant in combinations of midazolam and dexamethasone.[14]

Drug	Dose in syringe (mg)	Volume in syringe (ml)	Concentration (mg/ml)	Diluent	Outcome	Data Type
A	2800		11.20			
B	112	250	0.45	NaCl	✗[†]	LAB[11]
C	105		0.42			

[†]Infusion rate set at 1.5 ml/hour over the 7 days.

Tramadol (A), Haloperidol (B), and Hyoscine Butylbromide (C)

Summary: No problems with physical stability encountered.

Drug	Dose in syringe (mg)	Volume in syringe (ml)	Concentration (mg/ml)	Diluent	Outcome	Data Type
A	2800		11.20		✓(P)	
B	52.5	250	0.21	NaCl	(7 days)†	LAB[11]
C	420		1.68			

†Infusion rate set at 1.5 ml/hour over the 7 days.

Tramadol (A), Haloperidol (B), and Metoclopramide (C)

Summary: Although no problems with physical stability were encountered, the use of this combination of antiemetics is not generally recommended because of the increased risk of adverse effects.

Drug	Dose in syringe (mg)	Volume in syringe (ml)	Concentration (mg/ml)	Diluent	Outcome	Data Type
A	2800		11.20		✓(P)	
B	52.5	250	0.21	NaCl	(7 days)†	LAB[11]
C	280		1.12			

†Infusion rate set at 1.5 ml/hour over the 7 days.

Tramadol (A), Haloperidol (B), and Midazolam (C)

Summary: No problems with physical stability encountered.

Drug	Dose in syringe (mg)	Volume in syringe (ml)	Concentration (mg/ml)	Diluent	Outcome	Data Type
A	2800		11.20		✓(P)	
B	52.5	250	0.21	NaCl	(7 days)†	LAB[11]
C	105		0.42			

†Infusion rate set at 1.5 ml/hour over the 7 days.

Tramadol (A), Hyoscine Butylbromide (B), and Metoclopramide (C)

Summary: No problems with physical stability encountered. This is not a sensible combination of anti-emetics, since the pro-kinetic action of metoclopramide is inhibited by hyoscine. Higher doses of metoclopramide will be required to overcome this. However, use of this combination is acceptable if metoclopramide is used for its central dopamine antagonist properties, although haloperidol is the preferred choice.

Drug	Dose in syringe (mg)	Volume in syringe (ml)	Concentration (mg/ml)	Diluent	Outcome	Data Type
A	2800		11.20		✓ (P)	LAB[11]
B	420	250	1.68	NaCl	(7 days)[†]	
C	280		1.12			

[†]Infusion rate set at 1.5 ml/hour over the 7 days.

Tramadol (A), Hyoscine Butylbromide (B), and Midazolam (C)

Summary: No problems with physical stability encountered.

Drug	Dose in syringe (mg)	Volume in syringe (ml)	Concentration (mg/ml)	Diluent	Outcome	Data Type
A	2800		11.20		✓ (P)	LAB[11]
B	420	250	1.68	NaCl	(7 days)[†]	
C	105		0.42			

[†]Infusion rate set at 1.5 ml/hour over the 7 days.

Tramadol (A), Metoclopramide (B), and Midazolam (C)

Summary: No problems with physical stability encountered.

Drug	Dose in syringe (mg)	Volume in syringe (ml)	Concentration (mg/ml)	Diluent	Outcome	Data Type
A	2800		11.20		✓ (P)	LAB[11]
B	280	250	1.12	NaCl	(7 days)[†]	
C	105		0.42			

[†]Infusion rate set at 1.5 ml/hour over the 7 days.

Clonazepam (A), Haloperidol (B), and Metoclopramide (C)

Summary: Although no problems with physical stability were encountered, this combination of antiemetics is not recommended due to the increased risk of undesirable effects. Loss of clonazepam observed when infused via PVC tubing.[1] Minimize loss by using non-PVC tubing.

Drug	Dose in syringe (mg)	Volume in syringe (ml)	Concentration (mg/ml)	Diluent	Outcome	Data Type
A	4		0.24		✓ (P) (24 h)	
B	10	17	0.59	WFI		CLIN
C	30		1.76			

Clonazepam (A), Hyoscine Hydrobromide (B), and Metoclopramide (C)

Summary: No problems with physical stability encountered. This is not a sensible combination because the pro-kinetic action of metoclopramide is (theoretically) inhibited by hyoscine. Higher doses of metoclopramide will be required to overcome this. However, use of this combination is acceptable if metoclopramide is used for its central dopamine antagonist properties, although haloperidol is preferable. Loss of clonazepam observed when infused via PVC tubing.[1] Minimize loss by using non-PVC tubing.

Drug	Dose in syringe (mg)	Volume in syringe (ml)	Concentration (mg/ml)	Diluent	Outcome	Data Type
A	1		0.06		✓ (P) (24 h)	
B	1.2	16	0.08	WFI		CLIN
C	30		1.88			

Cyclizine (A), Dexamethasone (B), and Hyoscine Butylbromide (C)

Summary: No problems with physical stability encountered at concentrations below, although the mixture may exhibit concentration-dependent physical incompatibility. Dexamethasone is usually given as a subcutaneous bolus injection (depending upon volume of injection) or via a separate CSCI. However, if dexamethasone is to be mixed with other drugs, it should be the last constituent added to the maximally diluted syringe. There may be initial transient turbidity upon the addition of dexamethasone.

Drug	Dose in syringe (mg)	Volume in syringe (ml)	Concentration (mg/ml)	Diluent	Outcome	Data Type
A	150		8.82		✓(P)	
B	12	17	0.71	WFI	(24 h)	CLIN
C	40		2.35			

Cyclizine (A), Haloperidol (B), and Midazolam (C)

Summary: No problems with physical stability encountered.

Drug	Dose in syringe (mg)	Volume in syringe (ml)	Concentration (mg/ml)	Diluent	Outcome	Data Type
A	150		8.82		✓(P)	
B	5	17	0.29	WFI	(24 h)	CLIN
C	30		1.76			
A	150		8.82		✓(P)	
B	10	17	0.59	WFI	(24 h)	CLIN
C	40		2.35			

Dexamethasone (A), Haloperidol (B), and Hyoscine Butylbromide (C)

Summary: Physically incompatible at these concentrations. Dexamethasone is usually given as a subcutaneous bolus injection (depending upon volume of injection) or via a separate CSCI. However, if dexamethasone is to be mixed with other drugs, it should be the last constituent added to the maximally diluted syringe. There may be initial transient turbidity upon the addition of dexamethasone.

Drug	Dose in syringe (mg)	Volume in syringe (ml)	Concentration (mg/ml)	Diluent	Outcome	Data Type
A	80		1.30			
B	37.5	60	0.63	NaCl	☒[†]	LAB[11]
C	300		5.00			

[†]Infusion rate set at 0.5 ml/hour over the 5 days.

Dexamethasone (A), Haloperidol (B), and Metoclopramide (C)

Summary: Physically incompatible at these concentrations. Dexamethasone is usually given as a subcutaneous bolus injection (depending upon volume of injection) or via a separate CSCI. However, if dexamethasone is to be mixed with other drugs, it should be the last constituent added to the maximally diluted syringe. There may be initial transient turbidity upon the addition of dexamethasone.

Drug	Dose in syringe (mg)	Volume in syringe (ml)	Concentration (mg/ml)	Diluent	Outcome	Data Type
A	80		1.33			
B	37.5	60	0.63	NaCl	☒[†]	LAB[11]
C	200		3.33			

[†]Infusion rate set at 0.5 ml/hour over the 5 days.

Dexamethasone (A), Haloperidol (B), and Midazolam (C)

Summary: Problems with physical stability may be concentration dependent. Dexamethasone is usually given as a subcutaneous bolus injection (depending upon volume of injection) or via a separate CSCI. However, if dexamethasone is to be mixed with other drugs, it should be the last constituent added to the maximally diluted syringe. There may be initial transient turbidity upon the addition of dexamethasone. Laboratory study suggests possibility of loss of midazolam at higher temperature (37° C) which may be significant in combinations of midazolam and dexamethasone.[14]

Drug	Dose in syringe (mg)	Volume in syringe (ml)	Concentration (mg/ml)	Diluent	Outcome	Data Type
A	8		0.44		✓ (P) (24 h)	CLIN
B	2.5	18	0.14	WFI		
C	2.5		0.14			
A	80		1.33		✗[†]	LAB[11]
B	37.5	60	0.63	NaCl		
C	75		1.25			

[†]Infusion rate set at 0.5 ml/hour over the 5 days.

Dexamethasone (A), Hyoscine Butylbromide (B), and Metoclopramide (C)

Summary: No problems with physical stability encountered. Dexamethasone is usually given as a subcutaneous bolus injection (depending upon volume of injection) or via a separate CSCI. However, if dexamethasone is to be mixed with other drugs, it should be the last constituent added to the maximally diluted syringe. There may be initial transient turbidity upon the addition of dexamethasone. This is not a sensible combination of antiemetics, since the pro-kinetic action of metoclopramide is (theoretically) inhibited by hyoscine. Higher doses of metoclopramide will be required to overcome this. However, use of this combination is acceptable if metoclopramide is used for its central dopamine antagonist properties.

Drug	Dose in syringe (mg)	Volume in syringe (ml)	Concentration (mg/ml)	Diluent	Outcome	Data Type
A	112		0.45		✓ (P)	
B	420	250	1.68	NaCl	(7 days)[†]	LAB[11]
C	280		1.12			

[†]Infusion rate set at 0.5 ml/hour over the 7 days.

Dexamethasone (A), Hyoscine Butylbromide (B), and Midazolam (C)

Summary: Physically incompatible at these concentrations. Dexamethasone is usually given as a subcutaneous bolus injection (depending upon volume of injection) or via a separate CSCI. However, if dexamethasone is to be mixed with other drugs, it should be the last constituent added to the maximally diluted syringe. There may be initial transient turbidity upon the addition of dexamethasone. Laboratory study suggests possibility of loss of midazolam at higher temperature (37° C) which may be significant in combinations of midazolam and dexamethasone.[14]

Drug	Dose in syringe (mg)	Volume in syringe (ml)	Concentration (mg/ml)	Diluent	Outcome	Data Type
A	8		0.80			
B	20	10	2.00	NaCl	☒	CLIN
C	5		0.50			
A	8		0.40			
B	20	20	1.00	WFI	☒	CLIN
C	10		0.50			
A	80		1.33			
B	300	60	5.00	NaCl	☒[†]	LAB[11]
C	75		1.25			

[†]Infusion rate set at 0.5 ml/hour over the 5 days.

Dexamethasone (A), Metoclopramide (B), and Midazolam (C)

Summary: Physically incompatible at these concentrations. Dexamethasone is usually given as a subcutaneous bolus injection (depending upon volume of injection) or via a separate CSCI. However, if dexamethasone is to be mixed with other drugs, it should be the last constituent added to the maximally diluted syringe. There may be initial transient turbidity upon the addition of dexamethasone. Laboratory study suggests possibility of loss of midazolam at higher temperature (37° C) which may be significant in combinations of midazolam and dexamethasone.[14]

Drug	Dose in syringe (mg)	Volume in syringe (ml)	Concentration (mg/ml)	Diluent	Outcome	Data Type
A	112		0.45			
B	280	250	1.12	NaCl	✗[†]	LAB[11]
C	105		0.42			

[†]Infusion rate set at 1.5 ml/hour over the 7 days.

Glycopyrronium (A), Levomepromazine (B) and Octreotide (C)

Summary: No problems with physical stability encountered. To avoid irritation at the site of infusion, levomepromazine may be given as a subcutaneous bolus injection at doses below 50 mg (= 2 ml).

Drug	Dose in syringe (mg)	Volume in syringe (ml)	Concentration (mg/ml)	Diluent	Outcome	Data Type
A	1.6		0.10		✓(P)	
B	12.5	16	0.78	WFI	(24 h)	CLIN
C	0.6		0.04			
A	1.6		0.09		✓(P)	
B	25	17	1.47	WFI	(24 h)	CLIN
C	0.6		0.04			
A	2.4		0.12		✓(P)	
B	25	20	1.25	NaCl	(24 h)	CLIN
C	1.0		0.05			
A	2.4		0.14		✓(P)	
B	18.75	17	1.10	NaCl	(24 h)	CLIN
C	0.5		0.03			

Haloperidol (A), Hyoscine Butylbromide (B), and Midazolam (C)

Summary: No problems with physical stability encountered.

Drug	Dose in syringe (mg)	Volume in syringe (ml)	Concentration (mg/ml)	Diluent	Outcome	Data Type
A	5		0.30		✓ (P)	
B	180	16.5	10.91	WFI	(24 h)	CLIN
C	10		0.61			
A	37.5		0.63		✓ (P)	
B	300	60	5.00	NaCl	(5 days)[†]	LAB[11]
C	75		1.25			

[†]Infusion rate set at 0.5 ml/hour over the 5 days.

Hyoscine Butylbromide (A), Levomepromazine (B), and Octreotide (C)

Summary: No problems with physical stability encountered. To avoid irritation at the site of infusion, levomepromazine may be given as a subcutaneous bolus injection at doses below 50 mg (= 2 ml).

Drug	Dose in syringe (mg)	Volume in syringe (ml)	Concentration (mg/ml)	Diluent	Outcome	Data Type
A	180		8.57		✓ (P)	
B	18.75	21	0.89	NaCl	(24 h)	CLIN
C	0.5		0.02			

Hyoscine Butylbromide (A), Metoclopramide (B), and Midazolam (C)

Summary: No problems with physical stability encountered. This is not a sensible combination of antiemetics, since the pro-kinetic action of metoclopramide is (theoretically) inhibited by hyoscine. Higher doses of metoclopramide will be required to overcome this. However, use of this combination is acceptable if metoclopramide is used for its central dopamine antagonist properties, although haloperidol is the preferred choice.

Drug	Dose in syringe (mg)	Volume in syringe (ml)	Concentration (mg/ml)	Diluent	Outcome	Data Type
A	300		5.00		✓ (P)	
B	200	60	3.33	NaCl	(5 days)[†]	LAB[11]
C	75		1.25			

[†]Infusion rate set at 0.5 ml/hour over the 5 days.

Hyoscine Hydrobromide (A), Ketorolac (B), and Ranitidine (C)

Summary: No problems with physical stability encountered.

Drug	Dose in syringe (mg)	Volume in syringe (ml)	Concentration (mg/ml)	Diluent	Outcome	Data Type
A	0.8		0.04		✓ (P)	
B	90	20	4.50	NaCl	(24 h)	CLIN
C	150		7.50			

Hyoscine Hydrobromide (A), Levomepromazine (B), and Midazolam (C)

Summary: No problems with physical stability encountered. To avoid irritation at the site of infusion, levomepromazine may be given as a subcutaneous bolus injection at doses below 50 mg (= 2ml).

Drug	Dose in syringe (mg)	Volume in syringe (ml)	Concentration (mg/ml)	Diluent	Outcome	Data Type
A	2.4		0.14		✓ (P)	
B	50	17	2.94	WFI	(24 h)	CLIN
C	40		2.35			

Levomepromazine (A), Metoclopramide (B), and Octreotide (C)

Summary: Although no problems with physical stability were encountered, the use of levomepromazine and metoclopramide is not generally recommended because of the increased risk of undesirable effects. Levomepromazine also antagonizes the prokinetic effect of metoclopramide. To avoid irritation at the site of infusion, levomepromazine may be given as a subcutaneous bolus injection at doses below 50 mg (= 2 ml).

Drug	Dose in syringe (mg)	Volume in syringe (ml)	Concentration (mg/ml)	Diluent	Outcome	Data Type
A	6.25		0.42		✓ (P)	
B	60	15	4.00	WFI	(12 h)	CLIN
C	0.3		0.02			

Levomepromazine (A), Midazolam (B), and Octreotide (C)

Summary: No problems with physical stability encountered. To avoid irritation at the site of infusion, levomepromazine may be given as a subcutaneous bolus injection at doses below 50 mg (= 2 ml).

Drug	Dose in syringe (mg)	Volume in syringe (ml)	Concentration (mg/ml)	Diluent	Outcome	Data Type
A	12.5		0.83		✓ (P)	
B	20	15	1.33	NaCl	(24 h)	CLIN
C	0.6		0.04			
A	37.5		2.21		✓ (P)	
B	40	17	2.35	NaCl	(24 h)	CLIN
C	0.6		0.04			

Levomepromazine (A), Octreotide (B), and Ondansetron (C)

Summary: No problems with physical stability encountered. To avoid irritation at the site of infusion, levomepromazine may be given as a subcutaneous bolus injection at doses below 50 mg (= 2 ml).

Drug	Dose in syringe (mg)	Volume in syringe (ml)	Concentration (mg/ml)	Diluent	Outcome	Data Type
A	12.5		0.74		✓ (P)	
B	0.5	17	0.03	NaCl	(24 h)	CLIN
C	24		1.41			
A	25		1.12		✓ (P)	
B	0.6	21	0.38	NaCl	(24 h)	CLIN
C	24		2.31			

Compatibility data tables

Four Drugs

Drug A	B	C	D	Page
Alfentanil	Clonazepam	Dexamethasone	Haloperidol	232
Alfentanil	Clonazepam	Glycopyrronium	Haloperidol	232
Alfentanil	Cyclizine	Glycopyrronium	Haloperidol	233
Alfentanil	Cyclizine	Glycopyrronium	Midazolam	233
Alfentanil	Cyclizine	Haloperidol	Midazolam	234
Alfentanil	Cyclizine	Haloperidol	Octreotide	234
Alfentanil	Cyclizine	Haloperidol	Ondansetron	234
Alfentanil	Cyclizine	Levomepromazine	Midazolam	235
Alfentanil	Dexamethasone	Haloperidol	Midazolam	236
Alfentanil	Glycopyrronium	Levomepromazine	Midazolam	237
Alfentanil	Hyoscine Butylbromide	Levomepromazine	Octreotide	238
Alfentanil	Levomepromazine	Octreotide	Ondansetron	238
Diamorphine	Clonazepam	Cyclizine	Glycopyrronium	239
Diamorphine	Clonazepam	Cyclizine	Haloperidol	239
Diamorphine	Clonazepam	Dexamethasone	Haloperidol	240
Diamorphine	Clonazepam	Dexamethasone	Hyoscine Hydrobromide	241
Diamorphine	Clonazepam	Glycopyrronium	Haloperidol	242
Diamorphine	Clonazepam	Glycopyrronium	Levomepromazine	242
Diamorphine	Clonazepam	Haloperidol	Hyoscine Butylbromide	243
Diamorphine	Clonazepam	Haloperidol	Hyoscine Hydrobromide	243
Diamorphine	Clonazepam	Haloperidol	Levomepromazine	244
Diamorphine	Clonazepam	Hyoscine Butylbromide	Levomepromazine	244
Diamorphine	Clonazepam	Hyoscine Butylbromide	Midazolam	245
Diamorphine	Clonazepam	Hyoscine Butylbromide	Octreotide	245
Diamorphine	Clonazepam	Hyoscine Hydrobromide	Levomepromazine	246
Diamorphine	Cyclizine	Dexamethasone	Haloperidol	247

Drug A	B	C	D	Page
Diamorphine	Cyclizine	Dexamethasone	Hyoscine Hydrobromide	248
Diamorphine	Cyclizine	Dexamethasone	Metoclopramide	249
Diamorphine	Cyclizine	Glycopyrronium	Haloperidol	250
Diamorphine	Cyclizine	Glycopyrronium	Midazolam	251
Diamorphine	Cyclizine	Haloperidol	Hyoscine Butylbromide	252
Diamorphine	Cyclizine	Haloperidol	Hyoscine Hydrobromide	252
Diamorphine	Cyclizine	Haloperidol	Midazolam	253
Diamorphine	Cyclizine	Haloperidol	Octreotide	253
Diamorphine	Cyclizine	Hyoscine Butylbromide	Midazolam	254
Diamorphine	Cyclizine	Hyoscine Hydrobromide	Metoclopramide	254
Diamorphine	Cyclizine	Hyoscine Hydrobromide	Midazolam	255
Diamorphine	Cyclizine	Midazolam	Ranitidine	256
Diamorphine	Dexamethasone	Haloperidol	Hyoscine Butylbromide	256
Diamorphine	Dexamethasone	Haloperidol	Levomepromazine	257
Diamorphine	Dexamethasone	Haloperidol	Metoclopramide	258
Diamorphine	Dexamethasone	Hyoscine Hydrobromide	Midazolam	259
Diamorphine	Glycopyrronium	Haloperidol	Midazolam	260
Diamorphine	Glycopyrronium	Levomepromazine	Midazolam	261
Diamorphine	Glycopyrronium	Levomepromazine	Octreotide	262
Diamorphine	Glycopyrronium	Metoclopramide	Midazolam	263
Diamorphine	Glycopyrronium	Midazolam	Ondansetron	263
Diamorphine	Glycopyrronium	Octreotide	Ondansetron	264
Diamorphine	Haloperidol	Hyoscine Butylbromide	Levomepromazine	264
Diamorphine	Haloperidol	Hyoscine Butylbromide	Octreotide	265
Diamorphine	Haloperidol	Levomepromazine	Midazolam	265
Diamorphine	Haloperidol	Octreotide	Ondansetron	266
Diamorphine	Hyoscine Butylbromide	Levomepromazine	Midazolam	266
Diamorphine	Hyoscine Butylbromide	Levomepromazine	Octreotide	267
Diamorphine	Hyoscine Butylbromide	Levomepromazine	Ondansetron	268
Diamorphine	Hyoscine Butylbromide	Levomepromazine	Ranitidine	268

Drug A	B	C	D	Page
Diamorphine	Hyoscine Butylbromide	Octreotide	Ondansetron	269
Diamorphine	Hyoscine Hydrobromide	Levomepromazine	Midazolam	269
Diamorphine	Hyoscine Hydrobromide	Levomepromazine	Octreotide	270
Diamorphine	Levomepromazine	Metoclopramide	Octreotide	270
Diamorphine	Levomepromazine	Midazolam	Octreotide	271
Diamorphine	Levomepromazine	Octreotide	Ondansetron	271
Diamorphine	Midazolam	Octreotide	Ranitidine	272
Dihydrocodeine	Cyclizine	Haloperidol	Glycopyrronium	272
Dihydrocodeine	Cyclizine	Haloperidol	Midazolam	272
Hydromorphone	Cyclizine	Haloperidol	Midazolam	273
Hydromorphone	Glycopyrronium	Haloperidol	Promethazine	273
Hydromorphone	Glycopyrronium	Haloperidol	Octreotide	273
Hydromorphone	Glycopyrronium	Metoclopramide	Octreotide	274
Hydromorphone	Haloperidol	Hyoscine Hydrobromide	Promethazine	274
Hydromorphone	Hyoscine Hydrobromide	Metoclopramide	Octreotide	275
Hydromorphone	Ketamine	Metoclopramide	Midazolam	275
Morphine Hydrochloride	Dexamethasone	Haloperidol	Hyoscine Butylbromide	276
Morphine Hydrochloride	Dexamethasone	Haloperidol	Metoclopramide	276
Morphine Hydrochloride	Dexamethasone	Haloperidol	Midazolam	277
Morphine Hydrochloride	Dexamethasone	Hyoscine Butylbromide	Metoclopramide	278
Morphine Hydrochloride	Dexamethasone	Hyoscine Butylbromide	Midazolam	279
Morphine Hydrochloride	Dexamethasone	Metoclopramide	Midazolam	279
Morphine Hydrochloride	Haloperidol	Hyoscine Butylbromide	Metoclopramide	280
Morphine Hydrochloride	Haloperidol	Hyoscine Butylbromide	Midazolam	280
Morphine Hydrochloride	Hyoscine Butylbromide	Metoclopramide	Midazolam	281
Morphine Sulphate	Clonazepam	Cyclizine	Haloperidol	281
Morphine Sulphate	Clonazepam	Dexamethasone	Midazolam	282
Morphine Sulphate	Dexamethasone	Haloperidol	Octreotide	283
Morphine Sulphate	Dexamethasone	Hyoscine Hydrobromide	Midazolam	284
Morphine Sulphate	Glycopyrronium	Haloperidol	Promethazine	284

Drug A	B	C	D	Page
Morphine Sulphate	Glycopyrronium	Haloperidol	Octreotide	285
Morphine Sulphate	Glycopyrronium	Metoclopramide	Octreotide	285
Morphine Sulphate	Haloperidol	Hyoscine Hydrobromide	Promethazine	286
Morphine Sulphate	Hyoscine Hydrobromide	Metoclopramide	Octreotide	286
Morphine Sulphate	Ketamine	Metoclopramide	Midazolam	286
Morphine Tartrate	Clonazepam	Haloperidol	Midazolam	287
Morphine Tartrate	Cyclizine	Dexamethasone	Haloperidol	287
Morphine Tartrate	Cyclizine	Haloperidol	Midazolam	288
Morphine Tartrate	Cyclizine	Ketamine	Midazolam	288
Morphine Tartrate	Haloperidol	Ketamine	Midazolam	288
Morphine Tartrate	Ketamine	Metoclopramide	Midazolam	289
Oxycodone	Clonazepam	Haloperidol	Hyoscine Butylbromide	290
Oxycodone	Clonazepam	Hyoscine Butylbromide	Levomepromazine	290
Oxycodone	Clonazepam	Hyoscine Hydrobromide	Levomepromazine	291
Oxycodone	Haloperidol	Hyoscine Butylbromide	Midazolam	291
Oxycodone	Hyoscine Butylbromide	Levomepromazine	Midazolam	292
Oxycodone	Hyoscine Butylbromide	Levomepromazine	Octreotide	292
Oxycodone	Hyoscine Hydrobromide	Levomepromazine	Octreotide	293
Oxycodone	Levomepromazine	Octreotide	Ondansetron	293
Tramadol	Dexamethasone	Haloperidol	Hyoscine Butylbromide	294
Tramadol	Dexamethasone	Haloperidol	Metoclopramide	294
Tramadol	Dexamethasone	Haloperidol	Midazolam	295
Tramadol	Dexamethasone	Hyoscine Butylbromide	Metoclopramide	296
Tramadol	Dexamethasone	Hyoscine Butylbromide	Midazolam	297
Tramadol	Dexamethasone	Metoclopramide	Midazolam	297
Tramadol	Haloperidol	Hyoscine Butylbromide	Metoclopramide	298
Tramadol	Haloperidol	Hyoscine Butylbromide	Midazolam	298
Tramadol	Hyoscine Butylbromide	Metoclopramide	Midazolam	299
Cyclizine	Glycopyrronium	Haloperidol	Octreotide	299
Cyclizine	Glycopyrronium	Haloperidol	Ranitidine	300
Cyclizine	Glycopyrronium	Levomepromazine	Ranitidine	300
Dexamethasone	Haloperidol	Hyoscine Butylbromide	Midazolam	301
Dexamethasone	Hyoscine Butylbromide	Metoclopramide	Midazolam	302
Glycopyrronium	Levomepromazine	Octreotide	Ondansetron	302

Alfentanil (A), Clonazepam (B), Dexamethasone (C), and Haloperidol (D)

Summary: No problems with physical stability encountered at concentrations below, although the mixture may exhibit concentration-dependent physical incompatibility. Loss of clonazepam observed when infused via PVC tubing.[1] Minimize loss by using non-PVC tubing. Dexamethasone should be given via a bolus subcutaneous injection (depending upon volume), or separate CSCI. However, if dexamethasone is to be mixed with other drugs, it should be the last constituent added to the maximally diluted syringe. There may be initial transient turbidity upon the addition of dexamethasone.

Drug	Dose in syringe (mg)	Volume in syringe (ml)	Concentration (mg/ml)	Diluent	Outcome	Data Type
A	2		0.12			
B	4	17	0.24	WFI	✓ (P) (24 h)	CLIN
C	16		0.94			
D	3		0.18			

Alfentanil (A), Clonazepam (B), Glycopyrronium (C), and Haloperidol (D)

Summary: No problems with physical stability encountered. Loss of clonazepam observed when infused via PVC tubing.[1] Minimize loss by using non-PVC tubing.

Drug	Dose in syringe (mg)	Volume in syringe (ml)	Concentration (mg/ml)	Diluent	Outcome	Data Type
A	3		0.20			
B	2	15	0.13	WFI	✓ (P) (24 h)	CLIN
C	0.8		0.05			
D	5		0.33			

Alfentanil (A), Cyclizine (B), Glycopyrronium (C), and Haloperidol (D)

Summary: No problems with physical stability encountered. Crystallization may occur as concentrations increase.

Drug	Dose in syringe (mg)	Volume in syringe (ml)	Concentration (mg/ml)	Diluent	Outcome	Data Type
A	2		0.12			
B	150	17	8.82	WFI	✓ (P) (24 h)	CLIN
C	0.8		0.05			
D	10		0.59			

Alfentanil (A), Cyclizine (B), Glycopyrronium (C), and Midazolam (D)

Summary: No problems with physical stability encountered. Crystallization may occur as concentrations increase.

Drug	Dose in syringe (mg)	Volume in syringe (ml)	Concentration (mg/ml)	Diluent	Outcome	Data Type
A	4		0.24			
B	150	17	8.82	WFI	✓ (P) (24 h)	CLIN
C	0.8		0.05			
D	10		0.59			
A	5		0.38			
B	100	13	7.69	WFI	✓ (P) (24 h)	CLIN
C	0.6		0.05			
D	10		0.77			

Alfentanil (A), Cyclizine (B), Haloperidol (C), and Midazolam (D)

Summary: No problems with physical stability encountered. Crystallization may occur as concentrations increase.

Drug	Dose in syringe (mg)	Volume in syringe (ml)	Concentration (mg/ml)	Diluent	Outcome	Data Type
A	5		0.24			
B	150	21	7.14	WFI	✓ (P) (24 h)	CLIN
C	10		0.48			
D	4		1.90			

Alfentanil (A), Cyclizine (B), Haloperidol (C), and Octreotide (D)

Summary: No problems with physical stability encountered. Crystallization may occur as concentrations increase.

Drug	Dose in syringe (mg)	Volume in syringe (ml)	Concentration (mg/ml)	Diluent	Outcome	Data Type
A	10		0.63			
B	150	16	9.38	WFI	✓ (P) (24 h)	CLIN
C	10		0.63			
D	0.6		0.04			

Alfentanil (A), Cyclizine (B), Haloperidol (C), and Ondansetron (D)

Summary: No problems with physical stability encountered. Crystallization may occur as concentrations increase.

Drug	Dose in syringe (mg)	Volume in syringe (ml)	Concentration (mg/ml)	Diluent	Outcome	Data Type
A	11		0.55			
B	150	20	7.50	WFI	✓ (P) (24 h)	CLIN
C	5		0.25			
D	16		0.80			

Alfentanil (A), Cyclizine (B), Levomepromazine (C), and Midazolam (D)

Summary: No problems with physical stability encountered. Crystallization may occur as concentrations increase. Note that it is generally not necessary to administer both cyclizine and levomepromazine. To avoid irritation at the site of infusion, levomepromazine may be given as a subcutaneous bolus injection at doses below 50 mg (= 2 ml).

Drug	Dose in syringe (mg)	Volume in syringe (ml)	Concentration (mg/ml)	Diluent	Outcome	Data Type
A	5		0.24			
B	150	21	7.14	WFI	✓ (P) (24 h)	CLIN
C	25		1.19			
D	50		2.38			
A	10		0.59			
B	150	17	8.82	WFI	✓ (P) (24 h)	CLIN
C	12.5		0.74			
D	30		1.76			

Alfentanil (A), Dexamethasone (B), Haloperidol (C), and Midazolam (D)

Summary: This mixture exhibits concentration-dependent physical incompatibility. Dexamethasone should be given via a bolus subcutaneous injection (depending upon volume), or separate CSCI. However, if dexamethasone is to be mixed with other drugs, it should be the last constituent added to the maximally diluted syringe. There may be initial transient turbidity upon the addition of dexamethasone. Laboratory evidence suggests the possibility of loss of midazolam at a higher temperature (37° C) which may be significant in combinations of midazolam and dexamethasone[19].

Drug	Dose in syringe (mg)	Volume in syringe (ml)	Concentration (mg/ml)	Diluent	Outcome	Data Type
A	2		0.10			
B	1	21	0.05	WFI	✓ (P) (24 h)	CLIN
C	5		0.24			
D	20		0.95			
A	4.5		0.26			
B	16	17	0.94	WFI	☒	CLIN
C	3		0.18			
D	20		1.18			

Alfentanil (A), Glycopyrronium (B), Levomepromazine (C), and Midazolam (D)

Summary: No problems with physical stability encountered. To avoid irritation at the site of infusion, levomepromazine may be given as a subcutaneous bolus injection at doses below 50 mg (= 2 ml).

Drug	Dose in syringe (mg)	Volume in syringe (ml)	Concentration (mg/ml)	Diluent	Outcome	Data Type
A	2		0.06			
B	1.2	16	0.08	WFI	✓ (P)	CLIN
C	25		1.56		(24 h)	
D	20		1.25			
A	4		0.19			
B	1.2	21	0.06	NaCl	✓ (P)	CLIN
C	100		4.76		(12 h)	
D	25		1.19			
A	6		0.29			
B	1.2	21	0.06	NaCl	✓ (P)	CLIN
C	100		4.76		(12 h)	
D	35		1.67			
A	10.5		0.50			
B	0.8	21	0.04	NaCl	✓ (P)	CLIN
C	25		1.19		(24 h)	
D	50		2.38			
A	40		2.35			
B	1.0	17	0.06	NaCl	✓ (P)	CLIN
C	6.25		0.37		(12 h)	
D	12.5		0.74			

Alfentanil (A), Hyoscine Butylbromide (B), Levomepromazine (C), and Octreotide (D)

Summary: No problems with physical stability encountered. To avoid irritation at the site of infusion, levomepromazine may be given as a subcutaneous bolus injection at doses below 50 mg (= 2 ml).

Drug	Dose in syringe (mg)	Volume in syringe (ml)	Concentration (mg/ml)	Diluent	Outcome	Data Type
A	3		0.14			
B	240	21	11.43	NaCl	✓ (P) (24 h)	CLIN
C	12.5		0.60			
D	1.00		0.05			
A	8		0.47			
B	120	17	7.06	NaCl	✓ (P) (24 h)	CLIN
C	50		2.94			
D	0.6		0.04			
A	20		0.95			
B	180	21	8.57	NaCl	✓ (P) (24 h)	CLIN
C	37.5		1.79			
D	0.6		0.03			

Alfentanil (A), Levomepromazine (B), Octreotide (C), and Ondansetron (D)

Summary: No problems with physical stability encountered. To avoid irritation at the site of infusion, levomepromazine may be given as a subcutaneous bolus injection at doses below 50 mg (= 2 ml).

Drug	Dose in syringe (mg)	Volume in syringe (ml)	Concentration (mg/ml)	Diluent	Outcome	Data Type
A	6		0.35			
B	12.5	17	0.74	NaCl	✓ (P) (24 h)	CLIN
C	0.6		0.04			
D	24		1.41			

Diamorphine (A), Clonazepam (B), Cyclizine (C), and Glycopyrronium (D)

Summary: No problems with physical stability encountered. Loss of clonazepam observed when infused via PVC tubing.[1] Minimize loss by using non-PVC tubing.

Drug	Dose in syringe (mg)	Volume in syringe (ml)	Concentration (mg/ml)	Diluent	Outcome	Data Type
A	40		1.82			
B	6	22	0.27	WFI	✓ (P) (24 h)	CLIN
C	150		6.82			
D	2.4		0.11			
A	100		5.88			
B	4	17	0.24	WFI	✓ (P) (24 h)	CLIN
C	150		8.82			
D	1.2		0.07			

Diamorphine (A), Clonazepam (B), Cyclizine (C), and Haloperidol (D)

Summary: No problems with physical stability encountered. Crystallization may occur as concentrations increase. Loss of clonazepam observed when infused via PVC tubing.[1] Minimize loss by using non-PVC tubing.

Drug	Dose in syringe (mg)	Volume in syringe (ml)	Concentration (mg/ml)	Diluent	Outcome	Data Type
A	40		2.35			
B	2	17	0.12	WFI	✓ (P) (24 h)	CLIN
C	150		8.82			
D	5		0.29			

Diamorphine (A), Clonazepam (B), Dexamethasone (C), and Haloperidol (D)

Summary: No problems with physical stability encountered at concentrations below, although the mixture may exhibit concentration-dependent physical incompatibility. Dexamethasone should be given via a bolus subcutaneous injection (depending upon volume), or separate CSCI. However, if dexamethasone is to be mixed with other drugs, it should be the last constituent added to the maximally diluted syringe. There may be initial transient turbidity upon the addition of dexamethasone. Alternatively, either haloperidol or clonazepam may be given by subcutaneous bolus injection. Loss of clonazepam observed when infused via PVC tubing.[1] Minimize loss by using non-PVC tubing.

Drug	Dose in syringe (mg)	Volume in syringe (ml)	Concentration (mg/ml)	Diluent	Outcome	Data Type
A	5		0.29			
B	2	17	0.12	WFI	✓ (P) (24 h)	CLIN
C	12		0.71			
D	5		0.29			

Diamorphine (A), Clonazepam (B), Dexamethasone (C), and Hyoscine Hydrobromide (D)

Summary: No problems with physical stability encountered at concentrations below, although the mixture may exhibit concentration-dependent physical incompatibility. Dexamethasone should be given via a bolus subcutaneous injection (depending upon volume), or separate CSCI. However, if dexamethasone is to be mixed with other drugs, it should be the last constituent added to the maximally diluted syringe. There may be initial transient turbidity upon the addition of dexamethasone. Alternatively, clonazepam can be given as a subcutaneous bolus injection, although the dose may make this impractical. Loss of clonazepam observed when infused via PVC tubing.[1] Minimize loss by using non-PVC tubing.

Drug	Dose in syringe (mg)	Volume in syringe (ml)	Concentration (mg/ml)	Diluent	Outcome	Data Type
A	20		1.18			
B	4	17	0.24	WFI	✓ (P) (24 h)	CLIN
C	8		0.47			
D	1.8		0.11			

Diamorphine (A), Clonazepam (B), Glycopyrronium (C), and Haloperidol (D)

Summary: No problems with physical stability encountered. Loss of clonazepam observed when infused via PVC tubing.[1] Minimize loss by using non-PVC tubing.

Drug	Dose in syringe (mg)	Volume in syringe (ml)	Concentration (mg/ml)	Diluent	Outcome	Data Type
A	130		7.65			
B	4	17	0.24	WFI	✓ (P) (24 h)	CLIN
C	0.4		0.02			
D	5		0.29			
A	120		12.00			
B	2	10	0.20	WFI	✓ (P) (24 h)	CLIN
C	0.8		0.08			
D	5		0.50			

Diamorphine (A), Clonazepam (B), Glycopyrronium (C), and Levomepromazine (D)

Summary: No problems with physical stability encountered. To avoid irritation at the site of infusion, levomepromazine may be given as a subcutaneous bolus injection at doses below 50 mg (= 2 ml). Loss of clonazepam observed when infused via PVC tubing.[1] Minimize loss by using non-PVC tubing.

Drug	Dose in syringe (mg)	Volume in syringe (ml)	Concentration (mg/ml)	Diluent	Outcome	Data Type
A	10		0.59			
B	2	17	0.12	WFI	✓ (P) (24 h)	CLIN
C	1.2		0.07			
D	25		1.47			
A	50		2.38			
B	4	21	0.19	NaCl	✓ (P) (24 h)	CLIN
C	2.4		0.11			
D	25		1.19			

Diamorphine (A), Clonazepam (B), Haloperidol (C), and Hyoscine Butylbromide (D)

Summary: No problems with physical stability encountered. Loss of clonazepam observed when infused via PVC tubing.[1] Minimize loss by using non-PVC tubing.

Drug	Dose in syringe (mg)	Volume in syringe (ml)	Concentration (mg/ml)	Diluent	Outcome	Data Type
A	10		0.59			
B	2	17	0.12	WFI	✓ (P) (24 h)	CLIN
C	5		0.29			
D	80		4.71			
A	25		1.47			
B	2	17	0.12	NaCl	✓ (P) (24 h)	CLIN
C	5		0.29			
D	60		3.53			
A	90		5.29			
B	4	17	0.24	NaCl	✓ (P) (24 h)	CLIN
C	5		0.29			
D	120		7.06			

Diamorphine (A), Clonazepam (B), Haloperidol (C), and Hyoscine Hydrobromide (D)

Summary: No problems with physical stability encountered. Loss of clonazepam observed when infused via PVC tubing.[1] Minimize loss by using non-PVC tubing.

Drug	Dose in syringe (mg)	Volume in syringe (ml)	Concentration (mg/ml)	Diluent	Outcome	Data Type
A	120		8.00			
B	6	15	0.40	WFI	✓ (P) (24 h)	CLIN
C	5		0.33			
D	1.2		0.08			

Diamorphine (A), Clonazepam (B), Haloperidol (C), and Levomepromazine (D)

Summary: No problems with physical stability encountered. To avoid irritation at the site of infusion, levomepromazine may be given as a subcutaneous bolus injection at doses below 50 mg (= 2 ml). Generally, haloperidol and levomepromazine should not be used together because of the increased risk of adverse effects. Loss of clonazepam observed when infused via PVC tubing.[1] Minimize loss by using non-PVC tubing.

Drug	Dose in syringe (mg)	Volume in syringe (ml)	Concentration (mg/ml)	Diluent	Outcome	Data Type
A	15		0.88			
B	1	17	0.06	WFI	✓ (P) (24 h)	CLIN
C	5		0.29			
D	12.5		0.74			
A	150		8.82			
B	4	17	0.24	NaCl	✓ (P) (24 h)	CLIN
C	5		0.29			
D	25		1.47			

Diamorphine (A), Clonazepam (B), Hyoscine Butylbromide (C), and Levomepromazine (D)

Summary: No problems with physical stability encountered. To avoid irritation at the site of infusion, levomepromazine may be given as a subcutaneous bolus injection at doses below 50 mg (= 2 ml). Loss of clonazepam observed when infused via PVC tubing.[1] Minimize loss by using non-PVC tubing.

Drug	Dose in syringe (mg)	Volume in syringe (ml)	Concentration (mg/ml)	Diluent	Outcome	Data Type
A	45		2.81			
B	1	16	0.06	WFI	✓ (P) (24 h)	CLIN
C	60		3.75			
D	25		1.56			

Diamorphine (A), Clonazepam (B), Hyoscine Butylbromide (C), and Midazolam (D)

Summary: No problems with physical stability encountered. Note there is generally no reason to use both clonazepam and midazolam. Loss of clonazepam observed when infused via PVC tubing.[1] Minimize loss by using non-PVC tubing.

Drug	Dose in syringe (mg)	Volume in syringe (ml)	Concentration (mg/ml)	Diluent	Outcome	Data Type
A	750		34.09			
B	1.5	22	0.07	WFI	✓ (P) (24 h)	CLIN
C	60		2.73			
D	12.5		0.57			
A	1800		102.86			
B	3	17.5	0.17	WFI	✓ (P) (24 h)	CLIN
C	120		6.86			
D	10		0.57			

Diamorphine (A), Clonazepam (B), Hyoscine Butylbromide (C), and Octreotide (D)

Summary: No problems with physical stability encountered. Loss of clonazepam observed when infused via PVC tubing.[1] Minimize loss by using non-PVC tubing.

Drug	Dose in syringe (mg)	Volume in syringe (ml)	Concentration (mg/ml)	Diluent	Outcome	Data Type
A	15		0.88			
B	1	17	0.06	NaCl	✓ (P) (24 h)	CLIN
C	60		3.53			
D	0.5		0.03			
A	60		3.33			
B	3	18	0.17	NaCl	✓ (P) (24 h)	CLIN
C	140		7.78			
D	0.3		0.02			

Diamorphine (A), Clonazepam (B), Hyoscine Hydrobromide (C), and Levomepromazine (D)

Summary: No problems with physical stability encountered. To reduce irritation at the site of infusion, levomepromazine may be given as a subcutaneous bolus injection at doses below 50 mg (= 2 ml). Loss of clonazepam observed when infused via PVC tubing.[1] Minimize loss by using non-PVC tubing.

Drug	Dose in syringe (mg)	Volume in syringe (ml)	Concentration (mg/ml)	Diluent	Outcome	Data Type
A	60		3.53			
B	4	17	0.24	WFI	✓ (P) (24 h)	CLIN
C	1.6		0.09			
D	50		2.94			
A	80		4.71			
B	2	17	0.12	NaCl	✓ (P) (24 h)	CLIN
C	1.2		0.07			
D	25		1.47			
A	220		10.48			
B	4	21	0.19	NaCl	✓ (P) (24 h)	CLIN
C	2.4		0.11			
D	75		3.57			

Diamorphine (A), Cyclizine (B), Dexamethasone (C), and Haloperidol (D)

Summary: No problems with physical stability encountered at concentrations below, although the mixture may exhibit concentration-dependent physical incompatibility. Dexamethasone should be given via a bolus subcutaneous injection (depending upon volume), or separate CSCI. However, if dexamethasone is to be mixed with other drugs, it should be the last constituent added to the maximally diluted syringe. There may be initial transient turbidity upon the addition of dexamethasone.

Drug	Dose in syringe (mg)	Volume in syringe (ml)	Concentration (mg/ml)	Diluent	Outcome	Data Type
A	40		2.35			
B	150	17	8.82	WFI	✓ (P)	CLIN
C	4		0.24		(24 h)	
D	5		0.29			
A	70		4.12			
B	150	17	8.82	WFI	✓ (P)	CLIN
C	8		0.47		(24 h)	
D	5		0.29			
A	40		5.00			
B	150	8	18.75	WFI	✓ (P)	CLIN
C	1		0.13		(24 h)	
D	5		0.63			
A	90		5.29			
B	150	17	8.82	WFI	✓ (P)	CLIN
C	8		0.47		(24 h)	
D	10		0.59			
A	450		26.47			
B	150	17	8.82	WFI	✓ (P)	CLIN
C	8		0.47		(24 h)	
D	5		0.29			

Diamorphine (A), Cyclizine (B), Dexamethasone (C), and Hyoscine Hydrobromide (D)

Summary: No problems with physical stability encountered at concentrations below, although the mixture may exhibit concentration-dependent physical incompatibility. Dexamethasone should be given via a bolus subcutaneous injection (depending upon volume), or separate CSCI. However, if dexamethasone is to be mixed with other drugs, it should be the last constituent added to the maximally diluted syringe. There may be initial transient turbidity upon the addition of dexamethasone.

Drug	Dose in syringe (mg)	Volume in syringe (ml)	Concentration (mg/ml)	Diluent	Outcome	Data Type
A	60		3.53			
B	150	17	8.82	WFI	✓ (P) (24 h)	CLIN
C	8		0.47			
D	1.8		0.11			

Diamorphine (A), Cyclizine (B), Dexamethasone (C), and Metoclopramide (D)

Summary: This combination exhibits concentration-dependent physical incompatibility. Crystallization may occur as doses of metoclopramide and diamorphine increase relative to cyclizine. This is NOT a sensible combination of antiemetics, since the pro-kinetic action of metoclopramide may (theoretically) be inhibited by cyclizine. Higher doses of metoclopramide may be required to overcome this. However, use of this combination is acceptable if metoclopramide is used for its central dopamine antagonist properties, although haloperidol is the preferred choice. Dexamethasone should be given via a bolus subcutaneous injection (depending upon volume), or separate CSCI. However, if dexamethasone is to be mixed with other drugs, it should be the last constituent added to the maximally diluted syringe. There may be initial transient turbidity upon the addition of dexamethasone.

Drug	Dose in syringe (mg)	Volume in syringe (ml)	Concentration (mg/ml)	Diluent	Outcome	Data Type
A	50		2.94			
B	150	17	8.82	WFI	✓ (P)	CLIN
C	6		0.35		(24 h)	
D	30		1.76			
A	80		4.71			
B	150	17	8.82	WFI	✓ (P)	CLIN
C	2		0.12		(24 h)	
D	30		1.76			
A	190		11.88			
B	150	16	9.38	WFI	☒	CLIN
C	4		0.25			
D	30		1.88			
A	240		14.12			
B	150	17	8.82	WFI	☒	CLIN
C	4		0.24			
D	30		1.76			

Diamorphine (A), Cyclizine (B), Glycopyrronium (C), and Haloperidol (D)

Summary: No problems with physical stability encountered, although crystallization may occur as concentrations increase.

Drug	Dose in syringe (mg)	Volume in syringe (ml)	Concentration (mg/ml)	Diluent	Outcome	Data Type
A	120**		7.96			
B	150	17	8.82	–	✓ (P) (24 h)	CLIN
C	2.4		0.14			
D	10		0.59			
A	200		11.76			
B	150	17	8.82	WFI	✓ (P) (24 h)	CLIN
C	0.8		0.05			
D	5		0.29			

**Diamorphine reconstituted with glycopyrronium.

Diamorphine (A), Cyclizine (B), Glycopyrronium (C), Midazolam (D)

Summary: This combination may precipitate as concentrations increase. This mixture should be diluted maximally to overcome any problems.

Drug	Dose in syringe (mg)	Volume in syringe (ml)	Concentration (mg/ml)	Diluent	Outcome	Data Type
A	10		0.59			
B	150	17	8.82	WFI	✓ (P)	CLIN
C	1.6		0.09		(24 h)	
D	10		0.59			
A	10		0.5			
B	150	20	7.5	WFI	☒	CLIN
C	2.4		0.12			
D	15		0.75			
A	20		2.22			
B	150	9	16.67	WFI	☒	CLIN
C	0.6		0.07			
D	10		1.11			
A	100		6.67			
B	150	15	10.00	WFI	✓ (P)	CLIN
C	1.2		0.08		(24 h)	
D	20		1.33			

Diamorphine (A), Cyclizine (B), Haloperidol (C), and Hyoscine Butylbromide (D)

Summary: This mixture is likely to be physically incompatible. Crystallization may occur as concentrations increase. This can be overcome by substituting hyoscine butylbromide with glycopyrronium or hyoscine hydrobromide.

Drug	Dose in syringe (mg)	Volume in syringe (ml)	Concentration (mg/ml)	Diluent	Outcome	Data Type
A	60		3.53			
B	150	17	8.82	WFI	☒	CLIN
C	10		0.59			
D	80		4.71			
A	120		7.06			
B	75	17	4.41	WFI	✓ (P)	CLIN
C	2.5		0.15		(12 h)	
D	40		2.35			
A	320		18.82			
B	150	17	8.82	WFI	☒	CLIN
C	10		0.59			
D	120		7.06			

Diamorphine (A), Cyclizine (B), Haloperidol (C), and Hyoscine Hydrobromide (D)

Summary: No problems with physical stability encountered, although crystallization may occur as concentrations increase.

Drug	Dose in syringe (mg)	Volume in syringe (ml)	Concentration (mg/ml)	Diluent	Outcome	Data Type
A	50		2.94			
B	150	17	8.82	WFI	✓ (P)	CLIN
C	5		0.29		(24 h)	
D	2.4		0.14			
A	230		13.53			
B	150	17	8.82	WFI	✓ (P)	CLIN
C	10		0.59		(24 h)	
D	1.6		0.09			

Diamorphine (A), Cyclizine (B), Haloperidol (C), and Midazolam (D)

Summary: No problems with physical stability encountered, although crystallization may occur as concentrations increase.

Drug	Dose in syringe (mg)	Volume in syringe (ml)	Concentration (mg/ml)	Diluent	Outcome	Data Type
A	50		3.57			
B	150	17	10.71	WFI	✓ (P) (24 h)	CLIN
C	5		0.36			
D	20		1.43			
A	120		0.76			
B	150	17	10.71	WFI	✓ (P) (24 h)	CLIN
C	5		0.36			
D	10		0.59			
A	240		14.12			
B	150	17	8.82	WFI	✓ (P) (24 h)	CLIN
C	10		0.59			
D	30		1.76			

Diamorphine (A), Cyclizine (B), Haloperidol (C), and Octreotide (D)

Summary: No problems with physical stability encountered, although crystallization may occur as concentrations increase.

Drug	Dose in syringe (mg)	Volume in syringe (ml)	Concentration (mg/ml)	Diluent	Outcome	Data Type
A	30		1.76			
B	150	17	8.82	WFI	✓ (P) (24 h)	CLIN
C	10		0.59			
D	0.6		0.04			
A	130		1.76			
B	150	20	7.50	WFI	✓ (P) (24 h)	CLIN
C	10		0.50			
D	0.6		0.03			

Diamorphine (A), Cyclizine (B), Hyoscine Butylbromide (C), and Midazolam (D)

Summary: This mixture has been shown to be physically incompatible. The problem can be overcome by substituting hyoscine butylbromide with glycopyrronium or hyoscine hydrobromide.

Drug	Dose in syringe (mg)	Volume in syringe (ml)	Concentration (mg/ml)	Diluent	Outcome	Data Type
A	30		1.50			
B	150	20	7.50	WFI	☒	CLIN
C	100		5.00			
D	20		1.00			
A	150		8.82			
B	150	17	8.82	WFI	☒	CLIN
C	80		4.71			
D	20		1.18			

Diamorphine (A), Cyclizine (B), Hyoscine Hydrobromide (C), and Metoclopramide (D)

Summary: Crystallization is possible at higher concentrations. This mixture should be diluted maximally to overcome any problems. This is not a sensible combination because the pro-kinetic action of metoclopramide may (theoretically) be inhibited by cyclizine and hyoscine. Higher doses of metoclopramide will be required to overcome this. However, use of this combination is acceptable if metoclopramide is used for its central dopamine antagonist properties, although haloperidol is preferable.

Drug	Dose in syringe (mg)	Volume in syringe (ml)	Concentration (mg/ml)	Diluent	Outcome	Data Type
A	30		1.76			
B	150	17	8.82	WFI	✓ (P) (24 h)	CLIN
C	0.6		0.04			
D	30		1.76			
A	170		10.00			
B	150	20	8.82	WFI	✓ (P) (24 h)	CLIN
C	1.2		0.07			
D	30		1.76			

Diamorphine (A), Cyclizine (B), Hyoscine Hydrobromide (C), and Midazolam (D)

Summary: No problems with physical stability encountered, although crystallization may occur as concentrations increase.

Drug	Dose in syringe (mg)	Volume in syringe (ml)	Concentration (mg/ml)	Diluent	Outcome	Data Type
A	30		1.76			
B	150	17	8.82	WFI	✓ (P)	CLIN
C	1.2		0.07		(24 h)	
D	30		1.76			
A	40**		2.35			
B	150	17	8.82	–	✓ (P)	CLIN
C	2.4		0.14		(24 h)	
D	40		2.35			
A	45		2.65			
B	150	17	8.82	WFI	✓ (P)	CLIN
C	1.6		0.09		(24 h)	
D	30		1.76			
A	120		7.06			
B	150	17	8.82	WFI	✓ (P)	CLIN
C	1.6		0.09		(24 h)	
D	30		1.76			
A	160		8.00			
B	150	20	7.50	WFI	✓ (P)	CLIN
C	1.8		0.09		(24 h)	
D	50		2.50			

**Diamorphine reconstituted with midazolam.

Diamorphine (A), Cyclizine (B), Midazolam (C), and Ranitidine (D)

Summary: No problems with physical stability encountered, although crystallization/precipitation may occur as concentrations increase. Note that the mixture of midazolam and ranitidine alone exhibits concentration-dependent physical incompatibility.

Drug	Dose in syringe (mg)	Volume in syringe (ml)	Concentration (mg/ml)	Diluent	Outcome	Data Type
A	10		0.50			
B	150	20	7.50	WFI	✓ (P) (24 h)	CLIN
C	10		0.50			
D	150		7.50			

Diamorphine (A), Dexamethasone (B), Haloperidol (C), and Hyoscine Butylbromide (D)

Summary: No problems with physical stability encountered at concentrations below, although the mixture may exhibit concentration-dependent physical incompatibility. Dexamethasone should be given via a bolus subcutaneous injection (depending upon volume), or separate CSCI. However, if dexamethasone is to be mixed with other drugs, it should be the last constituent added to the maximally diluted syringe. There may be initial transient turbidity upon the addition of dexamethasone.

Drug	Dose in syringe (mg)	Volume in syringe (ml)	Concentration (mg/ml)	Diluent	Outcome	Data Type
A	70		4.12			
B	8	17	0.47	WFI	✓ (P) (24 h)	CLIN
C	5		0.29			
D	80		4.71			

Diamorphine (A), Dexamethasone (B), Haloperidol (C), and Levomepromazine (D)

Summary: Combination probably exhibits concentration-dependent physical incompatibility. Problem can be overcome by administering the dexamethasone via a bolus subcutaneous injection (depending upon volume), or separate CSCI. If dexamethasone is to be mixed with other drugs, it should be the last constituent added to the maximally diluted syringe. There may be initial transient turbidity upon the addition of dexamethasone. Levomepromazine and haloperidol should not generally be used together as this increases the risk of adverse effects. To reduce irritation at the site of infusion, levomepromazine may be given as a subcutaneous bolus injection at doses below 50 mg (= 2 ml).

Drug	Dose in syringe (mg)	Volume in syringe (ml)	Concentration (mg/ml)	Diluent	Outcome	Data Type
A	90		5.29			
B	6	17	0.35	WFI	☒	CLIN
C	10		0.59			
D	25		1.47			

Diamorphine (A), Dexamethasone (B), Haloperidol (C), and Metoclopramide (D)

Summary: Although no problems were encountered at these concentrations, the mixture is likely to exhibit concentration-dependent physical incompatibility. Metoclopramide and haloperidol should not generally be used together as this increases the risk of adverse effects. Dexamethasone should be given via a bolus subcutaneous injection (depending upon volume), or separate CSCI. However, if dexamethasone is to be mixed with other drugs, it should be the last constituent added to the maximally diluted syringe. There may be initial transient turbidity upon the addition of dexamethasone.

Drug	Dose in syringe (mg)	Volume in syringe (ml)	Concentration (mg/ml)	Diluent	Outcome	Data Type
A	120		7.06			
B	8	17	0.47	WFI	✓ (P) (24 h)	CLIN
C	10		0.59			
D	30		1.76			
A	260		15.29			
B	6	17	0.35	WFI	✓ (P) (24 h)	CLIN
C	5		0.29			
D	30		1.76			

Diamorphine (A), Dexamethasone (B), Hyoscine Hydrobromide (C), and Midazolam (D)

Summary: No problems with physical stability encountered at concentrations below, although the mixture may exhibit concentration-dependent physical incompatibility. Dexamethasone is usually given as a subcutaneous bolus injection (depending upon volume of injection) or via a separate CSCI. However, if dexamethasone is to be mixed with other drugs, it should be the last constituent added to the maximally diluted syringe. There may be initial transient turbidity upon the addition of dexamethasone. Note that laboratory evidence suggests the possibility of loss of midazolam at a higher temperature (37° C) which may be significant in combinations of midazolam and dexamethasone.[14]

Drug	Dose in syringe (mg)	Volume in syringe (ml)	Concentration (mg/ml)	Diluent	Outcome	Data Type
A	30		1.76			
B	4	17	0.24	WFI	✓ (P) (24 h)	CLIN
C	1.8		0.11			
D	15		0.88			
A	70		4.12			
B	8	17	0.47	WFI	✓ (P) (24 h)	CLIN
C	1.2		0.07			
D	30		1.76			
A	120		7.06			
B	8	17	0.47	WFI	✓ (P) (24 h)	CLIN
C	1.6		0.09			
D	20		1.18			

Diamorphine (A), Glycopyrronium (B), Haloperidol (C), and Midazolam (D)

Summary: No problems with physical stability encountered.

Drug	Dose in syringe (mg)	Volume in syringe (ml)	Concentration (mg/ml)	Diluent	Outcome	Data Type
A	10		0.63			
B	0.8	16	0.05	NaCl	✓ (P) (24 h)	CLIN
C	10		0.63			
D	20		1.25			
A	45		2.65			
B	1.2	17	0.07	WFI	✓ (P) (24 h)	CLIN
C	10		0.59			
D	20		1.18			
A	90		5.29			
B	0.8	17	0.05	WFI	✓ (P) (24 h)	CLIN
C	5		0.29			
D	30		1.76			
A	130		7.65			
B	1.6	17	0.09	WFI	✓ (P) (24 h)	CLIN
C	10		0.59			
D	20		1.18			

Diamorphine (A), Glycopyrronium (B), Levomepromazine (C), and Midazolam (D)

Summary: No problems with physical stability encountered. To avoid irritation at the site of infusion, levomepromazine may be given as a subcutaneous bolus injection at doses below 50 mg (= 2 ml).

Drug	Dose in syringe (mg)	Volume in syringe (ml)	Concentration (mg/ml)	Diluent	Outcome	Data Type
A	50		2.38		✓ (P) (24 h)	CLIN
B	1.8	21	0.09	WFI		
C	25		1.19			
D	50		2.38			
A	300**		14.29		✓ (P) (24 h)	CLIN
B	2.0	21	0.10	NaCl		
C	12.5		0.60			
D	25		1.19			

**Reconstituted with glycopyrronium.

Diamorphine (A), Glycopyrronium (B), Levomepromazine (C), and Octreotide (D)

Summary: No problems with physical stability encountered. To avoid irritation at the site of infusion, levomepromazine may be given as a subcutaneous bolus injection at doses below 50 mg (= 2 ml).

Drug	Dose in syringe (mg)	Volume in syringe (ml)	Concentration (mg/ml)	Diluent	Outcome	Data Type
A	15		0.88			
B	1.8	17	0.11	NaCl	✓ (P) (24 h)	CLIN
C	12.5		0.74			
D	0.3		0.02			
A	20		1.18			
B	1.8	17	0.11	WFI	✓ (P) (24 h)	CLIN
C	50		2.94			
D	0.6		0.04			
A	40		2.00			
B	1.6	20	0.08	WFI	✓ (P) (24 h)	CLIN
C	12.5		0.63			
D	0.6		0.03			
A	100		5.88			
B	2.4	17	0.14	WFI	✓ (P) (24 h)	CLIN
C	50		2.94			
D	0.6		0.04			
A	190		9.50			
B	2.4	20	0.12	WFI	✓ (P) (24 h)	CLIN
C	25		1.25			
D	0.5		0.03			

Diamorphine (A), Glycopyrronium (B), Metoclopramide (C), and Midazolam (D)

Summary: No problems with physical stability encountered.

Drug	Dose in syringe (mg)	Volume in syringe (ml)	Concentration (mg/ml)	Diluent	Outcome	Data Type
A	40**		2.35			
B	1.2	20	0.07	–	✓ (P) (24 h)	CLIN
C	40		2.35			
D	30		1.76			

**Diamorphine reconstituted with glycopyrronium.

Diamorphine (A), Glycopyrronium (B), Midazolam (C), and Ondansetron (D)

Summary: No problems with physical stability encountered.

Drug	Dose in syringe (mg)	Volume in syringe (ml)	Concentration (mg/ml)	Diluent	Outcome	Data Type
A	20		0.95			
B	1.2	21	0.06	NaCl	✓ (P) (24 h)	CLIN
C	20		0.95			
D	16		0.76			

Diamorphine (A), Glycopyrronium (B), Octreotide (C), and Ondansetron (D)

Summary: No problems with physical stability encountered.

Drug	Dose in syringe (mg)	Volume in syringe (ml)	Concentration (mg/ml)	Diluent	Outcome	Data Type
A	10**		0.50			
B	1.8	20	0.09	–	✓ (P) (24 h)	CLIN
C	0.3		0.02			
D	16		0.80			
A	120		7.06			
B	1.2	17	0.07	NaCl	✓ (P) (24 h)	CLIN
C	0.5		0.03			
D	12		0.71			

**Diamorphine reconstituted with glycopyrronium.

Diamorphine (A), Haloperidol (B), Hyoscine Butylbromide (C), and Levomepromazine (D)

Summary: No problems with physical stability encountered. Note that it is not usually necessary to give both haloperidol and levomepromazine together. To prevent site irritation, levomepromazine may be given as a subcutaneous injection at doses below 50 mg (= 2 ml).

Drug	Dose in syringe (mg)	Volume in syringe (ml)	Concentration (mg/ml)	Diluent	Outcome	Data Type
A	40		2.35			
B	10	17	0.59	WFI	✓ (P) (24 h)	CLIN
C	80		4.71			
D	25		1.47			

Diamorphine (A), Haloperidol (B), Hyoscine Butylbromide (C), and Octreotide (D)

Summary: No problems with physical stability encountered.

Drug	Dose in syringe (mg)	Volume in syringe (ml)	Concentration (mg/ml)	Diluent	Outcome	Data Type
A	55		2.50			
B	5	22	0.23	NaCl	✓ (P) (24 h)	CLIN
C	240		10.91			
D	0.3		0.01			
A	180		10.59			
B	5	17	0.29	NaCl	✓ (P) (24 h)	CLIN
C	100		5.88			
D	0.5		0.03			

Diamorphine (A), Haloperidol (B), Levomepromazine (C), and Midazolam (D)

Summary: No problems with physical stability encountered. Note that it is normally not necessary to use haloperidol and levomepromazine together. To avoid irritation at the site of infusion, levomepromazine may be given as a subcutaneous bolus injection at doses below 50 mg (= 2 ml).

Drug	Dose in syringe (mg)	Volume in syringe (ml)	Concentration (mg/ml)	Diluent	Outcome	Data Type
A	25		1.47			
B	5	17	0.29	NaCl	✓ (P) (24 h)	CLIN
C	25		1.47			
D	15		0.88			
A	130		7.65			
B	5	17	0.29	NaCl	✓ (P) (24 h)	CLIN
C	37.5		2.21			
D	40		2.35			
A	320		18.82			
B	10	17	0.59	WFI	✓ (P) (24 h)	CLIN
C	150		8.82			
D	20		1.18			

Diamorphine (A), Haloperidol (B), Octreotide (C), and Ondansetron (D)

Summary: No problems with physical stability encountered.

Drug	Dose in syringe (mg)	Volume in syringe (ml)	Concentration (mg/ml)	Diluent	Outcome	Data Type
A	5		0.23			
B	5	22	0.23	NaCl	✓ (P) (24 h)	CLIN
C	0.3		0.01			
D	32		1.45			

Diamorphine (A), Hyoscine Butylbromide (B), Levomepromazine (C), and Midazolam (D)

Summary: No problems with physical stability encountered. To avoid irritation at the site of infusion, levomepromazine may be given as a subcutaneous bolus injection at doses below 50 mg (= 2 ml).

Drug	Dose in syringe (mg)	Volume in syringe (ml)	Concentration (mg/ml)	Diluent	Outcome	Data Type
A	15		0.88			
B	120	17	7.06	WFI	✓ (P) (24 h)	CLIN
C	12.5		0.74			
D	25		1.47			
A	120		7.06			
B	80	17	4.71	WFI	✓ (P) (24 h)	CLIN
C	25		1.47			
D	20		1.18			
A	730		42.94			
B	90	17	5.29	WFI	✓ (P) (24 h)	CLIN
C	50		2.94			
D	10		0.59			

Diamorphine (A), Hyoscine Butylbromide (B), Levomepromazine (C), and Octreotide (D)

Summary: No problems with physical stability encountered. To avoid irritation at the site of infusion, levomepromazine may be given as a subcutaneous bolus injection at doses below 50 mg (= 2 ml).

Drug	Dose in syringe (mg)	Volume in syringe (ml)	Concentration (mg/ml)	Diluent	Outcome	Data Type
A	10		0.42			
B	180	24	7.50	NaCl	✓ (P) (24 h)	CLIN
C	12.5		0.52			
D	1.0		0.04			
A	40		2.35			
B	90	17	5.29	WFI	✓ (P) (24 h)	CLIN
C	25		1.47			
D	0.6		0.04			
A	50		2.94			
B	60	17	3.53	WFI	✓ (P) (24 h)	CLIN
C	50		2.94			
D	0.6		0.04			
A	70		3.18			
B	240	22	10.91	NaCl	✓ (P) (24 h)	CLIN
C	12.5		0.57			
D	0.3		0.01			
A	80		3.20			
B	160	25	6.40	NaCl	✓ (P) (24 h)	CLIN
C	18.75		0.75			
D	0.3		0.01			
A	60		3.53			
B	120	17	7.06	NaCl	✓ (P) (24 h)	CLIN
C	12.5		0.74			
D	0.3		0.02			

Diamorphine (A), Hyoscine Butylbromide (B), Levomepromazine (C), and Ondansetron (D)

Summary: No problems with physical stability encountered. To avoid irritation at the site of infusion, levomepromazine may be given as a subcutaneous bolus injection at doses below 50 mg (= 2 ml).

Drug	Dose in syringe (mg)	Volume in syringe (ml)	Concentration (mg/ml)	Diluent	Outcome	Data Type
A	60		2.73			
B	120	22	5.45	NaCl	✓ (P) (24 h)	CLIN
C	25		1.14			
D	16		0.73			
A	250		11.90			
B	180	21	8.57	WFI	✓ (P) (24 h)	CLIN
C	37.5		1.79			
D	16		0.76			

Diamorphine (A), Hyoscine Butylbromide (B), Levomepromazine (C), and Ranitidine (D)

Summary: No problems with physical stability encountered, although precipitation may occur as concentrations increase. Note that the mixture of levomepromazine and ranitidine alone exhibits concentration-dependent physical incompatibility. To avoid irritation at the site of infusion, levomepromazine may be given as a subcutaneous bolus injection at doses below 50 mg (= 2 ml).

Drug	Dose in syringe (mg)	Volume in syringe (ml)	Concentration (mg/ml)	Diluent	Outcome	Data Type
A	10		0.67			
B	120	15	8.00	WFI	✓ (P) (24 h)	CLIN
C	12.5		0.83			
D	150		10.00			

Diamorphine (A), Hyoscine Butylbromide (B), Octreotide (C), and Ondansetron (D)

Summary: No problems with physical stability encountered.

Drug	Dose in syringe (mg)	Volume in syringe (ml)	Concentration (mg/ml)	Diluent	Outcome	Data Type
A	35		1.67			
B	120	21	5.71	NaCl	✓ (P) (12 h)	CLIN
C	0.15		0.01			
D	8		0.38			
A	40		2.35			
B	60	17	3.53	WFI	✓ (P) (24 h)	CLIN
C	0.6		0.04			
D	16		0.94			

Diamorphine (A), Hyoscine Hydrobromide (B), Levomepromazine (C), and Midazolam (D)

Summary: No problems with physical stability encountered. To avoid irritation at the site of infusion, levomepromazine may be given as a subcutaneous bolus injection at doses below 50 mg (= 2 ml).

Drug	Dose in syringe (mg)	Volume in syringe (ml)	Concentration (mg/ml)	Diluent	Outcome	Data Type
A	35		2.80			
B	2.4	12.5	0.19	WFI	✓ (P) (24 h)	CLIN
C	12.5		1.00			
D	20		1.60			
A	700**		43.75			
B	2.4	17	0.15	NaCl	✓ (P) (24 h)	CLIN
C	12.5		0.78			
D	20		1.25			

**Reconstituted with 1 ml water for injections.

Diamorphine (A), Hyoscine Hydrobromide (B), Levomepromazine (C), and Octreotide (D)

Summary: No problems with physical stability encountered. To avoid irritation at the site of infusion, levomepromazine may be given as a subcutaneous bolus injection at doses below 50 mg (= 2 ml).

Drug	Dose in syringe (mg)	Volume in syringe (ml)	Concentration (mg/ml)	Diluent	Outcome	Data Type
A	20		1.25			
B	1.2	16	0.08	NaCl	✓ (P) (24 h)	CLIN
C	12.5		0.78			
D	0.3		0.02			

Diamorphine (A), Levomepromazine (B), Metoclopramide (C), and Octreotide (D)

Summary: No problems with physical stability encountered. This is NOT a sensible combination of antiemetics, since the pro-kinetic action of metoclopramide may (theoretically) be inhibited by levomepromazine. Higher doses of metoclopramide may be required to overcome this. In addition, there is an increased risk of adverse effects. To avoid irritation at the site of infusion, levomepromazine may be given as a subcutaneous bolus injection at doses below 50 mg (= 2 ml).

Drug	Dose in syringe (mg)	Volume in syringe (ml)	Concentration (mg/ml)	Diluent	Outcome	Data Type
A	2.5		0.17			
B	12.5	15	0.83	WFI	✓ (P) (24 h)	CLIN
C	30		2.00			
D	0.6		0.04			

Diamorphine (A), Levomepromazine (B), Midazolam (C), and Octreotide (D)

Summary: No problems with physical stability encountered. To avoid irritation at the site of infusion, levomepromazine may be given as a subcutaneous bolus injection at doses below 50 mg (= 2 ml).

Drug	Dose in syringe (mg)	Volume in syringe (ml)	Concentration (mg/ml)	Diluent	Outcome	Data Type
A	40		2.35			
B	12.5	17	0.74	WFI	✓ (P) (24 h)	CLIN
C	20		1.18			
D	0.5		0.03			

Diamorphine (A), Levomepromazine (B), Octreotide (C), and Ondansetron (D)

Summary: No problems with physical stability encountered. To avoid irritation at the site of infusion, levomepromazine may be given as a subcutaneous bolus injection at doses below 50 mg (= 2 ml).

Drug	Dose in syringe (mg)	Volume in syringe (ml)	Concentration (mg/ml)	Diluent	Outcome	Data Type
A	20		1.05			
B	25	19	1.32	NaCl	✓ (P) (24 h)	CLIN
C	0.3		0.02			
D	16		0.84			
A	15		1.07			
B	12.5	14	0.89	NaCl	✓ (P) (24 h)	CLIN
C	1.0		0.07			
D	16		1.14			
A	60		3.53			
B	12.5	17	0.74	NaCl	✓ (P) (24 h)	CLIN
C	0.6		0.04			
D	24		1.41			

Diamorphine (A), Midazolam (B), Octreotide (C), and Ranitidine (D)

Summary: No problems with physical stability encountered, although precipitation may occur as concentrations increase. Note that the mixture of midazolam and ranitidine alone exhibits concentration-dependent physical incompatibility.

Drug	Dose in syringe (mg)	Volume in syringe (ml)	Concentration (mg/ml)	Diluent	Outcome	Data Type
A	20		1.05			
B	15	19	0.79	NaCl	✓ (P) (24 h)	CLIN
C	0.6		0.03			
D	150		7.89			

Dihydrocodeine (A), Cyclizine (B), Haloperidol (C), and Glycopyrronium (D)

Summary: No problems with physical stability encountered.

Drug	Dose in syringe (mg)	Volume in syringe (ml)	Concentration (mg/ml)	Diluent	Outcome	Data Type
A	100		5.88			
B	150	17	8.82	WFI	✓ (P) (24 h)	CLIN
C	5		0.29			
D	0.8		0.05			

Dihydrocodeine (A), Cyclizine (B), Haloperidol (C), and Midazolam (D)

Summary: No problems with physical stability encountered.

Drug	Dose in syringe (mg)	Volume in syringe (ml)	Concentration (mg/ml)	Diluent	Outcome	Data Type
A	250		15.63			
B	150	16	9.38	WFI	✓ (P) (24 h)	CLIN
C	5		0.31			
D	20		1.25			

Hydromorphone (A), Cyclizine (B), Haloperidol (C), and Midazolam (D)

Summary: No problem with physical stability encountered.

Drug	Dose in syringe (mg)	Volume in syringe (ml)	Concentration (mg/ml)	Diluent	Outcome	Data Type
A	32		1.78			
B	300	18	16.67	WFI	✓ (P) (24 h)	CLIN
C	2		0.11			
D	10		0.56			

Hydromorphone (A), Glycopyrronium (B), Haloperidol (C), and Promethazine (D)

Summary: No problems with physical stability encountered, although haloperidol and promethazine should not normally be given together.

Drug	Dose in syringe (mg)	Volume in syringe (ml)	Concentration (mg/ml)	Diluent	Outcome	Data Type
A	250		12.50			
B	2.4	20	0.12	DEX	✓ (P) (24 h)	LAB
C	5		0.25			
D	100		5.00			

Hydromorphone (A), Glycopyrronium (B), Haloperidol (C), and Octreotide (D)

Summary: No problems with physical stability encountered.

Drug	Dose in syringe (mg)	Volume in syringe (ml)	Concentration (mg/ml)	Diluent	Outcome	Data Type
A	100		9.71			
B	1.2	10.3	0.12	DEX	✓ (P) (24 h)	LAB
C	10		0.97			
D	0.3		0.03			

Hydromorphone (A), Glycopyrronium (B), Metoclopramide (C), and Octreotide (D)

Summary: No problems with physical stability encountered. This is NOT a sensible combination of antiemetics, since the pro-kinetic action of metoclopramide is inhibited by glycopyrronium. Higher doses of metoclopramide will be required to overcome this. However, use of this combination is acceptable if metoclopramide is used for its central dopamine antagonist properties, although haloperidol is the preferred choice.

Drug	Dose in syringe (mg)	Volume in syringe (ml)	Concentration (mg/ml)	Diluent	Outcome	Data Type
A	100		6.99			
B	1.2	14.3	0.08	DEX	✓ (P) (24 h)	LAB
C	30		2.10			
D	0.3		0.02			

Hydromorphone (A), Haloperidol (B), Hyoscine Hydrobromide (C), and Promethazine (D)

Summary: Physically incompatible at these concentrations.

Drug	Dose in syringe (mg)	Volume in syringe (ml)	Concentration (mg/ml)	Diluent	Outcome	Data Type
A	100		12.50			
B	10	8	1.25	DEX	✗	LAB
C	1.2		0.15			
D	50		6.25			

Hydromorphone (A), Hyoscine Hydrobromide (B), Metoclopramide (C), and Octreotide (D)

Summary: No problems with physical stability encountered. This is NOT a sensible combination of antiemetics, since the pro-kinetic action of metoclopramide is inhibited by hyoscine. Higher doses of metoclopramide will be required to overcome this. However, use of this combination is acceptable if metoclopramide is used for its central dopamine antagonist properties, although haloperidol is the preferred choice.

Drug	Dose in syringe (mg)	Volume in syringe (ml)	Concentration (mg/ml)	Diluent	Outcome	Data Type
A	100		8.85			
B	1.2	11.3	0.11	DEX	✓ (P) (24 h)	LAB
C	30		2.65			
D	0.3		0.03			

Hydromorphone (A), Ketamine (B), Metoclopramide (C), and Midazolam (D)

Summary: No problem with physical stability encountered.

Drug	Dose in syringe (mg)	Volume in syringe (ml)	Concentration (mg/ml)	Diluent	Outcome	Data Type
A	50		2.78			
B	200	18	11.11	NaCl	✓ (P) (24 h)	CLIN
C	30		1.67			
D	5		0.28			

Morphine Hydrochloride (A), Dexamethasone (B), Haloperidol (C), and Hyoscine Butylbromide (D)

Summary: Physically incompatible at these concentrations. Dexamethasone is usually given as a subcutaneous bolus injection (depending upon volume of injection) or via a separate CSCI.

Drug	Dose in syringe (mg)	Volume in syringe (ml)	Concentration (mg/ml)	Diluent	Outcome	Data Type
A	420		1.68			
B	112	250	0.45	NaCl	☒[†]	LAB[11]
C	52.5		0.21			
D	420		1.68			

[†]Infusion rate set at 1.5 ml/hour over the 7 days.

Morphine Hydrochloride (A), Dexamethasone (B), Haloperidol (C), and Metoclopramide (D)

Summary: Physically incompatible at these concentrations. Dexamethasone is usually given as a subcutaneous bolus injection (depending upon volume of injection) or via a separate CSCI.

Drug	Dose in syringe (mg)	Volume in syringe (ml)	Concentration (mg/ml)	Diluent	Outcome	Data Type
A	420		1.68			
B	112	250	0.45	NaCl	☒[†]	LAB[11]
C	52.5		0.21			
D	280		1.12			

[†]Infusion rate set at 1.5 ml/hour over the 7 days.

Morphine Hydrochloride (A), Dexamethasone (B), Haloperidol (C), and Midazolam (D)

Summary: Physically incompatible at these concentrations. Laboratory study suggests possibility of loss of midazolam at higher temperature (37° C) which may be significant in combinations of midazolam and dexamethasone.[14] Dexamethasone is usually given as a subcutaneous bolus injection (depending upon volume of injection) or via a separate CSCI. However, if dexamethasone is to be mixed with other drugs, it should be the last constituent added to the maximally diluted syringe. There may be initial transient turbidity upon the addition of dexamethasone.

Drug	Dose in syringe (mg)	Volume in syringe (ml)	Concentration (mg/ml)	Diluent	Outcome	Data Type
A	420		1.68			
B	112	250	0.45	NaCl	✗[†]	LAB[11]
C	52.5		0.21			
D	105		0.42			

[†]Infusion rate set at 1.5 ml/hour over the 7 days.

Morphine Hydrochloride (A), Dexamethasone (B), Hyoscine Butylbromide (C), and Metoclopramide (D)

Summary: No problems with physical stability encountered. This is NOT a sensible combination of antiemetics, since the pro-kinetic action of metoclopramide may (theoretically) be inhibited by hyoscine. Higher doses of metoclopramide will be required to overcome this. However, use of this combination is acceptable if metoclopramide is used for its central dopamine antagonist properties, since haloperidol cannot be used. Dexamethasone is usually given as a subcutaneous bolus injection (depending upon volume of injection) or via a separate CSCI. However, if dexamethasone is to be mixed with other drugs, it should be the last constituent added to the maximally diluted syringe.

Drug	Dose in syringe (mg)	Volume in syringe (ml)	Concentration (mg/ml)	Diluent	Outcome	Data Type
A	420		1.68			
B	112	250	0.45	NaCl	✓ (P) (7 days)[†]	LAB[11]
C	420		1.68			
D	280		1.12			

[†]Infusion rate set at 1.5 ml/hour over the 7 days.

Morphine Hydrochloride (A), Dexamethasone (B), Hyoscine Butylbromide (C), and Midazolam (D)

Summary: Physically incompatible at these concentrations. Laboratory study suggests possibility of loss of midazolam at higher temperature (37° C) which may be significant in combinations of midazolam and dexamethasone.[14] Dexamethasone is usually given as a subcutaneous bolus injection (depending upon volume of injection) or via a separate CSCI. However, if dexamethasone is to be mixed with other drugs, it should be the last constituent added to the maximally diluted syringe. There may be initial transient turbidity upon the addition of dexamethasone.

Drug	Dose in syringe (mg)	Volume in syringe (ml)	Concentration (mg/ml)	Diluent	Outcome	Data Type
A	420		1.68			
B	112	250	0.45	NaCl	☒[†]	LAB[11]
C	420		1.68			
D	105		0.42			

[†]Infusion rate set at 1.5 ml/hour over the 7 days.

Morphine Hydrochloride (A), Dexamethasone (B), Metoclopramide (C), and Midazolam (D)

Summary: Physically incompatible at these concentrations. Dexamethasone is usually given as a subcutaneous bolus injection (depending upon volume of injection) or via a separate CSCI. However, if dexamethasone is to be mixed with other drugs, it should be the last constituent added to the maximally diluted syringe. There may be initial transient turbidity upon the addition of dexamethasone. Laboratory study suggests possibility of loss of midazolam at higher temperature (37° C) which may be significant in combinations of midazolam and dexamethasone.[14]

Drug	Dose in syringe (mg)	Volume in syringe (ml)	Concentration (mg/ml)	Diluent	Outcome	Data Type
A	420		1.68			
B	112	250	0.45	NaCl	☒[†]	LAB[11]
C	280		1.12			
D	105		0.42			

[†]Infusion rate set at 1.5 ml/hour over the 7 days.

Morphine Hydrochloride (A), Haloperidol (B), Hyoscine Butylbromide (C), and Metoclopramide (D)

Summary: No problems with physical stability encountered. This is NOT a sensible combination of antiemetics, since the pro-kinetic action of metoclopramide is inhibited by hyoscine. Higher doses of metoclopramide will be required to overcome this. In addition, the combination of haloperidol and metoclopramide is generally not recommended and will increase the risk of adverse effects.

Drug	Dose in syringe (mg)	Volume in syringe (ml)	Concentration (mg/ml)	Diluent	Outcome	Data Type
A	420		1.68			
B	52.5	250	0.21	NaCl	✓ (P) (7 days)[†]	LAB[11]
C	420		1.68			
D	280		0.12			

[†]Infusion rate set at 1.5 ml/hour over the 7 days.

Morphine Hydrochloride (A), Haloperidol (B), Hyoscine Butylbromide (C), and Midazolam (D)

Summary: No problems with physical stability encountered.

Drug	Dose in syringe (mg)	Volume in syringe (ml)	Concentration (mg/ml)	Diluent	Outcome	Data Type
A	420		1.68			
B	52.5	250	0.21	NaCl	✓ (P) (7 days)[†]	LAB[11]
C	420		1.68			
D	105		0.42			

[†]Infusion rate set at 1.5 ml/hour over the 7 days.

Morphine Hydrochloride (A), Hyoscine Butylbromide (B), Metoclopramide (C), and Midazolam (D)

Summary: No problems with physical stability encountered. This is NOT a sensible combination, since the pro-kinetic action of metoclopramide is inhibited by hyoscine. Higher doses of metoclopramide will be required to overcome this. However, use of this combination is acceptable if metoclopramide is used for its central dopamine antagonist properties, although haloperidol would be the preferred choice.

Drug	Dose in syringe (mg)	Volume in syringe (ml)	Concentration (mg/ml)	Diluent	Outcome	Data Type
A	420		1.68			
B	420	250	1.68	NaCl	✓ (P) (7 days)[†]	LAB[11]
C	280		1.12			
D	105		0.42			

[†]Infusion rate set at 1.5 ml/hour over the 7 days.

Morphine Sulphate (A), Clonazepam (B), Cyclizine (C), and Haloperidol (D)

Summary: No problems with physical stability encountered. Loss of clonazepam observed when infused via PVC tubing.[1] Minimize loss by using non-PVC tubing.

Drug	Dose in syringe (mg)	Volume in syringe (ml)	Concentration (mg/ml)	Diluent	Outcome	Data Type
A	10		0.56			
B	1	18	0.06	WFI	✓ (P) (24 h)	CLIN
C	100		5.56			
D	2.5		0.14			

Morphine Sulphate (A), Clonazepam (B), Dexamethasone (C), and Midazolam (D)

Summary: No problems with physical stability encountered at concentrations below, although the mixture may exhibit concentration-dependent physical incompatibility. Dexamethasone should be given via a bolus subcutaneous injection (depending upon volume), or separate CSCI. However, if dexamethasone is to be mixed with other drugs, it should be the last constituent added to the maximally diluted syringe. There may be initial transient turbidity upon the addition of dexamethasone. Laboratory study suggests possibility of loss of midazolam at higher temperature (37° C) which may be significant in combinations of midazolam and dexamethasone.[14] Loss of clonazepam observed when infused via PVC tubing.[1] Minimize loss by using non-PVC tubing.

Drug	Dose in syringe (mg)	Volume in syringe (ml)	Concentration (mg/ml)	Diluent	Outcome	Data Type
A	20		1.11			
B	4	18	0.22	WFI	✓ (P) (24 h)	CLIN
C	12		0.67			
D	10		0.56			

Morphine Sulphate (A), Dexamethasone (B), Haloperidol (C), and Octreotide (D)

Summary: No problems with physical stability encountered at concentrations below, although the mixture may exhibit concentration-dependent physical incompatibility. Dexamethasone is usually given as a subcutaneous bolus injection (depending upon volume of injection) or via a separate CSCI. However, if dexamethasone is to be mixed with other drugs, it should be the last constituent added to the maximally diluted syringe. There may be initial transient turbidity upon the addition of dexamethasone.

Drug	Dose in syringe (mg)	Volume in syringe (ml)	Concentration (mg/ml)	Diluent	Outcome	Data Type
A	30		1.67			
B	8	18	0.44	NaCl	✓ (P) (24 h)	CLIN
C	2.5		0.14			
D	0.2		0.01			
A	60		3.33			
B	8	18	0.44	NaCl	✓ (P) (24 h)	CLIN
C	5		0.28			
D	0.2		0.01			

Morphine Sulphate (A), Dexamethasone (B), Hyoscine Hydrobromide (C), and Midazolam (D)

Summary: No problems with physical stability encountered at concentrations below, although the mixture may exhibit concentration-dependent physical incompatibility. Dexamethasone should be given via a bolus subcutaneous injection (depending upon volume), or separate CSCI. However, if dexamethasone is to be mixed with other drugs, it should be the last constituent added to the maximally diluted syringe. There may be initial transient turbidity upon the addition of dexamethasone. Laboratory study suggests possibility of loss of midazolam at higher temperature (37° C) which may be significant in combinations of midazolam and dexamethasone.[19]

Drug	Dose in syringe (mg)	Volume in syringe (ml)	Concentration (mg/ml)	Diluent	Outcome	Data Type
A	30		1.67			
B	4	18	0.22	NaCl	✓ (P) (24 h)	CLIN
C	0.4		0.02			
D	15		0.83			
A	30		1.67			
B	4	18	0.22	NaCl	✓ (P) (24 h)	CLIN
C	0.8		0.04			
D	15		0.83			

Morphine Sulphate (A), Glycopyrronium (B), Haloperidol (C), and Promethazine (D)

Summary: No problems with physical stability encountered, although haloperidol and promethazine should not normally be given together.

Drug	Dose in syringe (mg)	Volume in syringe (ml)	Concentration (mg/ml)	Diluent	Outcome	Data Type
A	400		22.22			
B	2.4	18	0.13	DEX	✓ (P) (24 h)	LAB
C	5		0.28			
D	100		5.56			

Morphine Sulphate (A), Glycopyrronium (B), Haloperidol (C), and Octreotide (D)

Summary: No problems with physical stability encountered.

Drug	Dose in syringe (mg)	Volume in syringe (ml)	Concentration (mg/ml)	Diluent	Outcome	Data Type
A	400		24.54			
B	1.2	16.3	0.07	DEX	✓ (P) (24 h)	LAB
C	10		0.61			
D	0.3		0.02			

Morphine Sulphate (A), Glycopyrronium (B), Metoclopramide (C), and Octreotide (D)

Summary: No problems with physical stability encountered. However, this is NOT a sensible combination of antiemetics, since the pro-kinetic action of metoclopramide is inhibited by glycopyrronium. Higher doses of metoclopramide will be required to overcome this. However, use of this combination is acceptable if metoclopramide is used for its central dopamine antagonist properties, although haloperidol is the preferred choice.

Drug	Dose in syringe (mg)	Volume in syringe (ml)	Concentration (mg/ml)	Diluent	Outcome	Data Type
A	400		19.70			
B	1.2	20.3	0.06	DEX	✓ (P) (24 h)	LAB
C	30		1.48			
D	0.3		0.01			

Morphine Sulphate (A), Haloperidol (B), Hyoscine Hydrobromide (C), and Promethazine (D)

Summary: Physically incompatible at these concentrations.

Drug	Dose in syringe (mg)	Volume in syringe (ml)	Concentration (mg/ml)	Diluent	Outcome	Data Type
A	400		28.57			
B	10	14	0.71	DEX	☒	LAB
C	1.2		0.09			
D	50		3.57			

Morphine Sulphate (A), Hyoscine Hydrobromide (B), Metoclopramide (C), and Octreotide (D)

Summary: No problems with physical stability encountered. However, this is NOT a sensible combination of antiemetics, since the pro-kinetic action of metoclopramide is inhibited by glycopyrronium. Higher doses of metoclopramide will be required to overcome this. However, use of this combination is acceptable if metoclopramide is used for its central dopamine antagonist properties, although haloperidol is the preferred choice.

Drug	Dose in syringe (mg)	Volume in syringe (ml)	Concentration (mg/ml)	Diluent	Outcome	Data Type
A	400		23.12			
B	1.2	17.3	0.07	DEX	✓ (P) (24 h)	LAB
C	30		1.73			
D	0.3		0.02			

Morphine Sulphate (A), Ketamine (B), Metoclopramide (C), and Midazolam (D)

Summary: No problems with physical stability encountered.

Drug	Dose in syringe (mg)	Volume in syringe (ml)	Concentration (mg/ml)	Diluent	Outcome	Data Type
A	15		0.83			
B	75	18	4.17	NaCl	✓ (P) (24 h)	CLIN
C	30		1.67			
D	5		0.28			

Morphine Tartrate (A), Clonazepam (B), Haloperidol (C), and Midazolam (D)

Summary: No problems with physical stability encountered. Note that there is no reason to administer both benzodiazepines. Loss of clonazepam observed when infused via PVC tubing.[1] Minimize loss by using non-PVC tubing.

Drug	Dose in syringe (mg)	Volume in syringe (ml)	Concentration (mg/ml)	Diluent	Outcome	Data Type
A	120		6.67			
B	2	18	0.11	NaCl	✓ (P) (24 h)	CLIN
C	5		0.28			
D	10		0.56			

Morphine Tartrate (A), Cyclizine (B), Dexamethasone (C), and Haloperidol (D)

Summary: No problems with physical stability encountered at concentrations below, although the mixture may exhibit concentration-dependent physical incompatibility. Dexamethasone is usually given as a subcutaneous bolus injection (depending upon volume of injection) or via a separate CSCI. However, if dexamethasone is to be mixed with other drugs, it should be the last constituent added to the maximally diluted syringe. There may be initial transient turbidity upon the addition of dexamethasone.

Drug	Dose in syringe (mg)	Volume in syringe (ml)	Concentration (mg/ml)	Diluent	Outcome	Data Type
A	120		6.67			
B	150	18	8.33	WFI	✓ (P) (24 h)	CLIN
C	4		0.22			
D	5		0.28			

Morphine Tartrate (A), Cyclizine (B), Haloperidol (C), and Midazolam (D)

Summary: No problems with physical stability encountered.

Drug	Dose in syringe (mg)	Volume in syringe (ml)	Concentration (mg/ml)	Diluent	Outcome	Data Type
A	100		5.56			
B	200	18	11.11	WFI	✓ (P) (24 h)	CLIN
C	20		1.11			
D	10		0.56			

Morphine Tartrate (A), Cyclizine (B), Ketamine (C), and Midazolam (D)

Summary: No problems with physical stability encountered.

Drug	Dose in syringe (mg)	Volume in syringe (ml)	Concentration (mg/ml)	Diluent	Outcome	Data Type
A	720		40.00			
B	50	18	2.78	WFI	✓ (P) (24 h)	CLIN
C	100		5.56			
D	5		0.28			

Morphine Tartrate (A), Haloperidol (B), Ketamine (C), and Midazolam (D)

Summary: No problems with physical stability encountered.

Drug	Dose in syringe (mg)	Volume in syringe (ml)	Concentration (mg/ml)	Diluent	Outcome	Data Type
A	240		13.33			
B	2.5	18	0.14	NaCl	✓ (P) (24 h)	CLIN
C	200		11.11			
D	7.5		0.42			
A	320		17.78			
B	1	18	0.06	NaCl	✓ (P) (24 h)	CLIN
C	75		4.17			
D	2.5		0.14			

Morphine Tartrate (A), Ketamine (B), Metoclopramide (C), and Midazolam (D)

Summary: No problems with physical stability encountered.

Drug	Dose in syringe (mg)	Volume in syringe (ml)	Concentration (mg/ml)	Diluent	Outcome	Data Type
A	120		6.67			
B	100	18	5.56	NaCl	✓ (P) (24 h)	CLIN
C	30		1.67			
D	2.5		0.14			
A	180		10.00			
B	200	18	11.11	NaCl	✓ (P) (24 h)	CLIN
C	20		1.11			
D	5		0.28			
A	240		13.33			
B	50	18	2.78	NaCl	✓ (P) (24 h)	CLIN
C	30		1.67			
D	2.5		0.14			
A	240		13.33			
B	100	18	5.56	NaCl	✓ (P) (24 h)	CLIN
C	30		1.67			
D	2.5		0.14			
A	480		26.67			
B	100	18	5.56	NaCl	✓ (P) (24 h)	CLIN
C	20		1.11			
D	5		0.28			
A	600		33.33			
B	50	18	2.78	NaCl	✓ (P) (24 h)	CLIN
C	20		1.11			
D	5		0.28			

Oxycodone (A), Clonazepam (B), Haloperidol (C), and Hyoscine Butylbromide (D)

Summary: No problems with physical stability encountered. Loss of clonazepam observed when infused via PVC tubing.[1] Minimize loss by using non-PVC tubing.

Drug	Dose in syringe (mg)	Volume in syringe (ml)	Concentration (mg/ml)	Diluent	Outcome	Data Type
A	100		5.00			
B	2	20	0.10	WFI	✓ (P) (24 h)	LAB[12]
C	60		3.00			
D	10		0.50			
A	100		5.00			
B	2	20	0.10	NaCl	✓ (P) (24 h)	LAB[12]
C	60		3.00			
D	10		0.50			

Oxycodone (A), Clonazepam (B), Hyoscine Butylbromide (C), and Levomepromazine (D)

Summary: No problems with physical stability encountered. Loss of clonazepam observed when infused via PVC tubing.[1] Minimize loss by using non-PVC tubing. To avoid irritation at the site of infusion, levomepromazine may be given as a subcutaneous bolus injection at doses below 50 mg (= 2 ml).

Drug	Dose in syringe (mg)	Volume in syringe (ml)	Concentration (mg/ml)	Diluent	Outcome	Data Type
A	100		5.00			
B	2	20	0.10	WFI	✓ (P) (24 h)	LAB[12]
C	80		4.00			
D	25		1.25			
A	100		5.00			
B	2	20	0.10	NaCl	✓ (P) (24 h)	LAB[12]
C	80		4.00			
D	25		1.25			

Oxycodone (A), Clonazepam (B), Hyoscine Hydrobromide (C), and Levomepromazine (D)

Summary: No problems with physical stability encountered. Loss of clonazepam observed when infused via PVC tubing.[1] Minimize loss by using non-PVC tubing. To avoid irritation at the site of infusion, levomepromazine may be given as a subcutaneous bolus injection at doses below 50 mg (= 2 ml).

Drug	Dose in syringe (mg)	Volume in syringe (ml)	Concentration (mg/ml)	Diluent	Outcome	Data Type
A	100		5.00			
B	2	20	0.10	WFI	✓ (P) (24 h)	LAB[12]
C	1.2		0.06			
D	25		1.25			
A	100		5.00			
B	2	20	0.10	NaCl	✓ (P) (24 h)	LAB[12]
C	1.2		0.06			
D	25		1.25			

Oxycodone (A), Haloperidol (B), Hyoscine Butylbromide (C), and Midazolam (D)

Summary: No problems with physical stability encountered.

Drug	Dose in syringe (mg)	Volume in syringe (ml)	Concentration (mg/ml)	Diluent	Outcome	Data Type
A	100		5.00			
B	5	20	0.25	WFI	✓ (P) (24 h)	LAB[12]
C	60		3.00			
D	20		1.00			
A	100		5.00			
B	5	20	0.25	NaCl	✓ (P) (24 h)	LAB[12]
C	60		3.00			
D	25		1.00			

Oxycodone (A), Hyoscine Butylbromide (B), Levomepromazine (C), and Midazolam (D)

Summary: No problems with physical stability encountered. To avoid irritation at the site of infusion, levomepromazine may be given as a subcutaneous bolus injection at doses below 50 mg (= 2 ml).

Drug	Dose in syringe (mg)	Volume in syringe (ml)	Concentration (mg/ml)	Diluent	Outcome	Data Type
A	100		5.00			
B	60	20	3.00	WFI	✓ (P) (24 h)	LAB[12]
C	25		1.25			
D	20		1.00			
A	100		5.00			
B	60	20	3.00	NaCl	✓ (P) (24 h)	LAB[12]
C	25		1.25			
D	20		1.00			

Oxycodone (A), Hyoscine Butylbromide (B), Levomepromazine (C), and Octreotide (D)

Summary: No problems with physical stability encountered. To avoid irritation at the site of infusion, levomepromazine may be given as a subcutaneous bolus injection at doses below 50 mg (= 2 ml).

Drug	Dose in syringe (mg)	Volume in syringe (ml)	Concentration (mg/ml)	Diluent	Outcome	Data Type
A	100		5.00			
B	120	20	6.00	WFI	✓ (P) (24 h)	LAB[12]
C	25		1.25			
D	0.5		0.03			
A	100		5.00			
B	120	20	6.00	NaCl	✓ (P) (24 h)	LAB[12]
C	25		1.25			
D	0.5		0.03			

Oxycodone (A), Hyoscine Hydrobromide (B), Levomepromazine (C), and Octreotide (D)

Summary: No problems with physical stability encountered. To avoid irritation at the site of infusion, levomepromazine may be given as a subcutaneous bolus injection at doses below 50 mg (= 2 ml).

Drug	Dose in syringe (mg)	Volume in syringe (ml)	Concentration (mg/ml)	Diluent	Outcome	Data Type
A	100		5.00			
B	120	20	0.06	WFI	✓ (P) (24 h)	LAB[12]
C	25		1.25			
D	25		0.03			
A	0.5		5.00			
B	120	20	0.06	NaCl	✓ (P) (24 h)	LAB[12]
C	25		1.25			
D	0.5		0.03			

Oxycodone (A), Levomepromazine (B), Octreotide (C), and Ondansetron (D)

Summary: No problems with physical stability encountered. To avoid irritation at the site of infusion, levomepromazine may be given as a subcutaneous bolus injection at doses below 50 mg (= 2 ml).

Drug	Dose in syringe (mg)	Volume in syringe (ml)	Concentration (mg/ml)	Diluent	Outcome	Data Type
A	100		5.00			
B	25	20	1.25	WFI	✓ (P) (24 h)	LAB[12]
C	0.5		0.03			
D	12		0.60			
A	100		5.00			
B	25	20	1.25	NaCl	✓ (P) (24 h)	LAB[12]
C	0.5		0.03			
D	12		0.60			

Tramadol (A), Dexamethasone (B), Haloperidol (C), and Hyoscine Butylbromide (D)

Summary: Physically incompatible at these concentrations. Dexamethasone is usually given as a subcutaneous bolus injection (depending upon volume of injection) or via a separate CSCI. However, if dexamethasone is to be mixed with other drugs, it should be the last constituent added to the maximally diluted syringe. There may be initial transient turbidity upon the addition of dexamethasone.

Drug	Dose in syringe (mg)	Volume in syringe (ml)	Concentration (mg/ml)	Diluent	Outcome	Data Type
A	2800		11.20			
B	112	250	0.45	NaCl	☒ †	LAB[11]
C	52.5		0.21			
D	420		1.68			

†Infusion rate set at 1.5 ml/hour over the 7 days.

Tramadol (A), Dexamethasone (B), Haloperidol (C), and Metoclopramide (D)

Summary: Physically incompatible at these concentrations. Dexamethasone is usually given as a subcutaneous bolus injection (depending upon volume of injection) or via a separate CSCI. However, if dexamethasone is to be mixed with other drugs, it should be the last constituent added to the maximally diluted syringe. There may be initial transient turbidity upon the addition of dexamethasone.

Drug	Dose in syringe (mg)	Volume in syringe (ml)	Concentration (mg/ml)	Diluent	Outcome	Data Type
A	420		1.68			
B	112	250	0.45	NaCl	☒ †	LAB[11]
C	52.5		0.21			
D	420		1.68			

†Infusion rate set at 1.5 ml/hour over the 7 days.

Tramadol (A), Dexamethasone (B), Haloperidol (C), and Midazolam (D)

Summary: Physically incompatible at these concentrations. Dexamethasone is usually given as a subcutaneous bolus injection (depending upon volume of injection) or via a separate CSCI. However, if dexamethasone is to be mixed with other drugs, it should be the last constituent added to the maximally diluted syringe. There may be initial transient turbidity upon the addition of dexamethasone. Laboratory study suggests possibility of loss of midazolam at higher temperature (37°C) which may be significant in combinations of midazolam and dexamethasone.[14]

Drug	Dose in syringe (mg)	Volume in syringe (ml)	Concentration (mg/ml)	Diluent	Outcome	Data Type
A	2800		11.20			
B	112	250	0.45	NaCl	☒[†]	LAB[11]
C	52.5		0.21			
D	105		0.42			

[†]Infusion rate set at 1.5 ml/hour over the 7 days.

Tramadol (A), Dexamethasone (B), Hyoscine Butylbromide (C), and Metoclopramide (D)

Summary: No problems with physical stability encountered. This is not a sensible combination of antiemetics, since the pro-kinetic action of metoclopramide is (theoretically) inhibited by hyoscine. Higher doses of metoclopramide will be required to overcome this. However, use of this combination is acceptable if metoclopramide is used for its central dopamine antagonist properties. Dexamethasone is usually given as a subcutaneous bolus injection (depending upon volume of injection) or via a separate CSCI. However, if dexamethasone is to be mixed with other drugs, it should be the last constituent added to the maximally diluted syringe. There may be initial transient turbidity upon the addition of dexamethasone.

Drug	Dose in syringe (mg)	Volume in syringe (ml)	Concentration (mg/ml)	Diluent	Outcome	Data Type
A	2800		11.20			
B	112	250	0.45	NaCl	✓ (P) (7 days)[†]	LAB[11]
C	420		1.68			
D	280		1.12			

[†]Infusion rate set at 1.5 ml/hour over the 7 days.

Tramadol (A), Dexamethasone (B), Hyoscine Butylbromide (C), and Midazolam (D)

Summary: Physically incompatible at these concentrations. Dexamethasone is usually given as a subcutaneous bolus injection (depending upon volume of injection) or via a separate CSCI. However, if dexamethasone is to be mixed with other drugs, it should be the last constituent added to the maximally diluted syringe. There may be initial transient turbidity upon the addition of dexamethasone. Laboratory study suggests possibility of loss of midazolam at higher temperature (37° C) which may be significant in combinations of midazolam and dexamethasone.[14]

Drug	Dose in syringe (mg)	Volume in syringe (ml)	Concentration (mg/ml)	Diluent	Outcome	Data Type
A	2800		11.20			
B	112	250	0.45	NaCl	☒[†]	LAB[11]
C	420		1.68			
D	105		0.42			

[†]Infusion rate set at 1.5 ml/hour over the 7 days.

Tramdol (A), Dexamethasone (B), Metoclopramide (C), and Midazolam (D)

Summary: Physically incompatible at these concentrations. Laboratory study suggests possibility of loss of midazolam at higher temperature (37° C) which may be significant in combinations of midazolam and dexamethasone.[1] Dexamethasone is usually given as a subcutaneous bolus injection (depending upon volume of injection) or via a separate CSCI.

Drug	Dose in syringe (mg)	Volume in syringe (ml)	Concentration (mg/ml)	Diluent	Outcome	Data Type
A	2800		11.20			
B	112	250	0.45	NaCl	☒[†]	LAB[11]
C	280		1.12			
D	105		0.42			

[†]Infusion rate set at 1.5 ml/hour over the 7 days.

Tramadol (A), Haloperidol (B), Hyoscine Butylbromide (C), and Metoclopramide (D)

Summary: No problems with physical stability encountered. This is NOT a sensible combination of antiemetics, since the pro-kinetic action of metoclopramide is (theoretically) inhibited by hyoscine. Higher doses of metoclopramide will be required to overcome this. In addition, the combination of haloperidol and metoclopramide is generally not recommended and will increase the risk of adverse effects.

Drug	Dose in syringe (mg)	Volume in syringe (ml)	Concentration (mg/ml)	Diluent	Outcome	Data Type
A	2800		11.20			
B	52.5	250	0.21	NaCl	✓ (P) (7 days)[†]	LAB[11]
C	420		1.68			
D	280		1.12			

[†]Infusion rate set at 1.5 ml/hour over the 7 days.

Tramadol (A), Haloperidol (B), Hyoscine Butylbromide (C), and Midazolam (D)

Summary: No problems with physical stability encountered.

Drug	Dose in syringe (mg)	Volume in syringe (ml)	Concentration (mg/ml)	Diluent	Outcome	Data Type
A	2800		11.20			
B	52.5	250	0.21	NaCl	✓ (P) (7 days)[†]	LAB[11]
C	420		1.68			
D	105		0.42			

[†]Infusion rate set at 1.5 ml/hour over the 7 days.

Tramadol (A), Hyoscine Butylbromide (B), Metoclopramide (C), and Midazolam (D)

Summary: No problems with physical stability encountered. This is NOT a sensible combination, since the pro-kinetic action of metoclopramide is inhibited by hyoscine. Higher doses of metoclopramide will be required to overcome this. However, use of this combination is acceptable if metoclopramide is used for its central dopamine antagonist properties, although haloperidol would be the preferred choice.

Drug	Dose in syringe (mg)	Volume in syringe (ml)	Concentration (mg/ml)	Diluent	Outcome	Data Type
A	2800		11.20			
B	420	250	1.68	NaCl	✓ (P) (7 days)†	LAB[11]
C	280		1.12			
D	105		0.42			

†Infusion rate set at 1.5 ml/hour over the 7 days.

Cyclizine (A), Glycopyrronium (B), Haloperidol (C), and Octreotide (D)

Summary: No problems with physical stability encountered, although crystallization can occur as concentrations increase.

Drug	Dose in syringe (mg)	Volume in syringe (ml)	Concentration (mg/ml)	Diluent	Outcome	Data Type
A	150		7.50			
B	2.4	20	0.12	WFI	✓ (P) (24 h)	CLIN
C	10		0.50			
D	0.6		0.03			

Cyclizine (A), Glycopyrronium (B), Haloperidol (C), and Ranitidine (D)

Summary: No problems with physical stability encountered.

Drug	Dose in syringe (mg)	Volume in syringe (ml)	Concentration (mg/ml)	Diluent	Outcome	Data Type
A	150		8.82			
B	2.4	17	0.07	WFI	✓ (P) (24 h)	CLIN
C	5		0.29			
D	150		8.82			

Cyclizine (A), Glycopyrronium (B), Levomepromazine (C), and Ranitidine (D)

Summary: No problems with physical stability encountered, although crystallization or precipitation can occur as doses increase. Levomepromazine and ranitidine alone show concentration-dependent physical incompatibility. Note that cyclizine and levomepromazine generally should not be prescribed concurrently. To avoid irritation at the site of infusion, levomepromazine may be given as a subcutaneous injection at doses below 50 mg (= 2 ml).

Drug	Dose in syringe (mg)	Volume in syringe (ml)	Concentration (mg/ml)	Diluent	Outcome	Data Type
A	150		7.50			
B	1.2	20	0.12	WFI	✓ (P) (24 h)	CLIN
C	25		0.50			
D	150		0.03			

Dexamethasone (A), Haloperidol (B), Hyoscine Butylbromide (C), and Midazolam (D)

Summary: Physically incompatible at these concentrations. Dexamethasone is usually given as a subcutaneous bolus injection (depending upon volume of injection) or via a separate CSCI. However, if dexamethasone is to be mixed with other drugs, it should be the last constituent added to the maximally diluted syringe. There may be initial transient turbidity upon the addition of dexamethasone. Laboratory study suggests possibility of loss of midazolam at higher temperature (37° C) which may be significant in combinations of midazolam and dexamethasone.[14]

Drug	Dose in syringe (mg)	Volume in syringe (ml)	Concentration (mg/ml)	Diluent	Outcome	Data Type
A	112		0.45			
B	52.5	250	0.21	NaCl	☒[†]	LAB[11]
C	420		1.68			
D	105		0.42			

[†]Infusion rate set at 1.5 ml/hour over the 7 days.

Dexamethasone (A), Hyoscine Butylbromide (B), Metoclopramide (C), and Midazolam (D)

Summary: Physically incompatible at these concentrations. Nonetheless, this is NOT a sensible combination, since the pro-kinetic action of metoclopramide is (theoretically) inhibited by hyoscine. Dexamethasone is usually given as a subcutaneous bolus injection (depending upon volume of injection) or via a separate CSCI. However, if dexamethasone is to be mixed with other drugs, it should be the last constituent added to the maximally diluted syringe. There may be initial transient turbidity upon the addition of dexamethasone. Laboratory study suggests possibility of loss of midazolam at higher temperature (37° C) which may be significant in combinations of midazolam and dexamethasone.[14]

Drug	Dose in syringe (mg)	Volume in syringe (ml)	Concentration (mg/ml)	Diluent	Outcome	Data Type
A	112		0.45			
B	420	250	1.68	NaCl	✗ [†]	LAB[11]
C	280		1.12			
D	105		0.42			

[†]Infusion rate set at 1.5 ml/hour over the 7 days.

Glycopyrronium (A), Levomepromazine (B), Octreotide (C), and Ondansetron (D)

Summary: No problems with physical stability encountered. To avoid irritation at the site of infusion, levomepromazine may be given as a subcutaneous bolus injection at doses below 50 mg (= 2 ml).

Drug	Dose in syringe (mg)	Volume in syringe (ml)	Concentration (mg/ml)	Diluent	Outcome	Data Type
A	0.6		0.03			
B	25	22	1.14	NaCl	✓ (P) (24 h)	CLIN
C	0.6		0.03			
D	24		1.09			

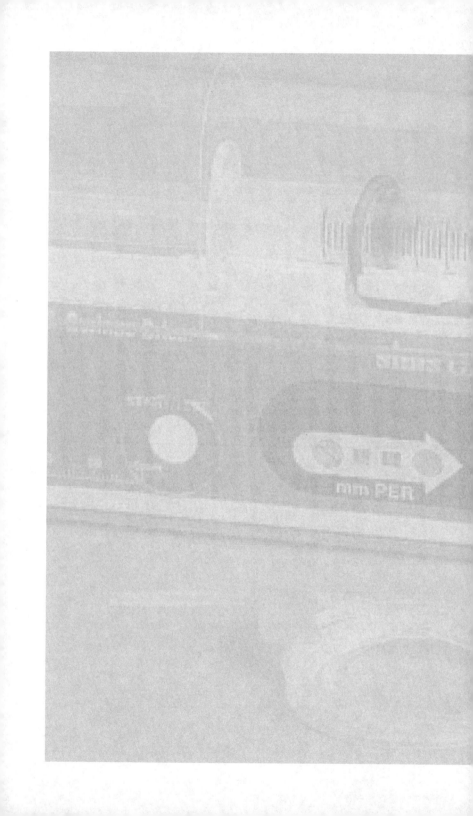

Compatibility data tables

Five Drugs

Drug A	B	C	D	E	Page
Alfentanil	Cyclizine	Haloperidol	Midazolam	Octreotide	306
Alfentanil	Glycopyrronium	Levomepromazine	Midazolam	Octreotide	306
Diamorphine	Clonazepam	Cyclizine	Dexamethasone	Haloperidol	307
Diamorphine	Clonazepam	Cyclizine	Glycopyrronium	Levomepromazine	307
Diamorphine	Clonazepam	Glycopyrronium	Levomepromazine	Octreotide	308
Diamorphine	Clonazepam	Hyoscine Butylbromide	Levomepromazine	Octreotide	308
Diamorphine	Cyclizine	Dexamethasone	Haloperidol	Midazolam	309
Diamorphine	Cyclizine	Glycopyrronium	Haloperidol	Midazolam	310
Diamorphine	Cyclizine	Glycopyrronium	Haloperidol	Octreotide	310
Diamorphine	Dexamethasone	Levomepromazine	Metoclopramide	Midazolam	311
Diamorphine	Glycopyrronium	Levomepromazine	Midazolam	Octreotide	312
Diamorphine	Glycopyrronium	Levomepromazine	Octreotide	Ondansetron	312
Diamorphine	Glycopyrronium	Midazolam	Octreotide	Ondansetron	313
Diamorphine	Haloperidol	Hyoscine Hydrobromide	Levomepromazine	Midazolam	313
Diamorphine	Hyoscine Butylbromide	Levomepromazine	Midazolam	Octreotide	314
Diamorphine	Hyoscine Butylbromide	Levomepromazine	Octreotide	Ondansetron	314
Diamorphine	Hyoscine Butylbromide	Midazolam	Octreotide	Ondansetron	315
Morphine Hydrochloride	Dexamethasone	Haloperidol	Hyoscine Butylbromide	Midazolam	315
Tramadol	Dexamethasone	Haloperidol	Hyoscine Butylbromide	Midazolam	316

Alfentanil (A), Cyclizine (B), Haloperidol (C), Midazolam (D), and Octreotide (E)

Summary: No problems with physical stability encountered, although crystallization may occur as concentrations increase.

Drug	Dose in syringe (mg)	Volume in syringe (ml)	Concentration (mg/ml)	Diluent	Outcome	Data Type
A	10		0.53			
B	150		7.89			
C	10	19	0.53	WFI	✓ (P) (24 h)	CLIN
D	20		1.05			
E	0.6		0.03			

Alfentanil (A), Glycopyrronium (B), Levomepromazine (C), Midazolam (D), and Octreotide (E)

Summary: No problems with physical stability encountered. To avoid irritation at the site of infusion, levomepromazine may be given as a subcutaneous bolus injection at doses below 50 mg (= 2 ml).

Drug	Dose in syringe (mg)	Volume in syringe (ml)	Concentration (mg/ml)	Diluent	Outcome	Data Type
A	3.5		0.19			
B	2.4		0.13			
C	6.25	18	0.35	WFI	✓ (P) (24 h)	CLIN
D	10		0.56			
E	0.6		0.03			

Diamorphine (A), Clonazepam (B), Cyclizine (C), Dexamethasone (D), and Haloperidol (E)

Summary: No problems with physical stability encountered at concentrations below, although the mixture may exhibit concentration-dependent physical incompatibility. Dexamethasone is usually given as a subcutaneous bolus injection (depending upon volume) or via a separate CSCI. However, if dexamethasone is to be mixed with other drugs, it should be the last constituent added to the maximally diluted syringe. There may be initial transient turbidity upon the addition of dexamethasone. Loss of clonazepam observed when infused via PVC tubing.[1] Minimize loss by using non-PVC tubing.

Drug	Dose in syringe (mg)	Volume in syringe (ml)	Concentration (mg/ml)	Diluent	Outcome	Data Type
A	50		3.33			
B	2		0.13		✓ (P)	
C	150	18	10.00	WFI		CLIN
D	1		0.07		(24 h)	
E	5		0.33			

Diamorphine (A), Clonazepam (B), Cyclizine (C), Glycopyrronium (D), and Levomepromazine (E)

Summary: No problems with stability. To avoid irritation at the site of infusion, levomepromazine may be given as a subcutaneous injection at doses below 50 mg (= 2 ml). Note that levomepromazine can be given as a bolus injection (less than 50 mg). Loss of clonazepam observed when infused via PVC tubing.[1] Minimize loss by using non-PVC tubing.

Drug	Dose in syringe (mg)	Volume in syringe (ml)	Concentration (mg/ml)	Diluent	Outcome	Data Type
A	50		3.33			
B	1.5		0.10		✓ (P)	
C	100	15	6.67	WFI		CLIN
D	1.8		0.12		(24 h)	
E	6.25		0.42			

Diamorphine (A), Clonazepam (B), Glycopyrronium (C), Levomepromazine (D), and Octreotide (E)

Summary: No problems with stability. To avoid irritation at the site of infusion, levomepromazine may be given as a subcutaneous injection at doses below 50 mg (= 2 ml). Note that levomepromazine can be given as a bolus injection (less than 50 mg). Loss of clonazepam observed when infused via PVC tubing.[1] Minimize loss by using non-PVC tubing.

Drug	Dose in syringe (mg)	Volume in syringe (ml)	Concentration (mg/ml)	Diluent	Outcome	Data Type
A	190		8.64			
B	1		0.05			
C	2.4	22	0.11	WFI	✓ (P) (24 h)	CLIN
D	25		1.14			
E	0.3		0.01			

Diamorphine (A), Clonazepam (B), Hyoscine Butylbromide (C), Levomepromazine (D), and Octreotide (E)

Summary: No problems with stability. To avoid irritation at the site of infusion, levomepromazine may be given as a subcutaneous injection at doses below 50 mg (= 2 ml). Note that levomepromazine can be given as a bolus injection (less than 50 mg). Loss of clonazepam observed when infused via PVC tubing.[1] Minimize loss by using non-PVC tubing.

Drug	Dose in syringe (mg)	Volume in syringe (ml)	Concentration (mg/ml)	Diluent	Outcome	Data Type
A	80		3.64			
B	3		0.14			
C	160	22	7.27	NaCl	✓ (P) (24 h)	CLIN
D	25		1.14			
E	0.3		0.01			

Diamorphine (A), Cyclizine (B), Dexamethasone (C), Haloperidol (D), and Midazolam (E)

Summary: No problems with physical stability encountered at concentrations below, although the mixture may exhibit concentration-dependent physical incompatibility. Dexamethasone is usually given as a subcutaneous bolus injection (depending upon volume of injection) or via a separate CSCI. However, if dexamethasone is to be mixed with other drugs, it should be the last constituent added to the maximally diluted syringe. There may be initial transient turbidity upon the addition of dexamethasone. Laboratory evidence suggests the possibility of loss of midazolam at a higher temperature (37° C) which may be significant in combinations of midazolam and dexamethasone.[14]

Drug	Dose in syringe (mg)	Volume in syringe (ml)	Concentration (mg/ml)	Diluent	Outcome	Data Type
A	130		15.29			
B	150		17.65		✓ (P)	
C	1	8.5	0.12	WFI	(24 h)	CLIN
D	5		0.59			
E	5		0.59			

Diamorphine (A), Cyclizine (B), Glycopyrronium (C), Haloperidol (D), and Midazolam (E)

Summary: No problems with physical stability encountered, although crystallization may occur as concentrations increase.

Drug	Dose in syringe (mg)	Volume in syringe (ml)	Concentration (mg/ml)	Diluent	Outcome	Data Type
A	20		1.18			
B	150		8.82			
C	0.8	17	0.05	WFI	✓ (P) (24 h)	CLIN
D	10		0.59			
E	25		1.47			
A	40		2.35			
B	150		8.82			
C	0.8	17	0.05	WFI	✓ (P) (24 h)	CLIN
D	5		0.29			
E	15		0.88			
A	140		6.36			
B	150		6.82			
C	1.6	22	0.07	WFI	✓ (P) (24 h)	CLIN
D	10		0.45			
E	40		1.82			

Diamorphine (A), Cyclizine (B), Glycopyrronium (C), Haloperidol (D), and Octreotide (E)

Summary: No problems with physical stability encountered although crystallization may occur as concentrations increase.

Drug	Dose in syringe (mg)	Volume in syringe (ml)	Concentration (mg/ml)	Diluent	Outcome	Data Type
A	40		2.35			
B	150		8.82			
C	1.8	17	0.11	WFI	✓ (P) (24 h)	CLIN
D	5		0.29			
E	0.6		0.04			

Diamorphine (A), Dexamethasone (B), Levomepromazine (C), Metoclopramide (D), and Midazolam (E)

Summary: No problems with physical stability encountered at concentrations below, although the mixture may exhibit concentration-dependent physical incompatibility. Dexamethasone should be given via a bolus subcutaneous injection (depending upon volume), or separate CSCI. However, if dexamethasone is to be mixed with other drugs, it should be the last constituent added to the maximally diluted syringe. There may be initial transient turbidity upon the addition of dexamethasone. Metoclopramide and levomepromazine should not generally be used together as this increases the risk of undesirable effects and levomepromazine may (theoretically) inhibit the prokinetic effect of metoclopramide. To reduce irritation at the site of infusion, levomepromazine may be given as a subcutaneous bolus injection at doses below 50 mg (= 2 ml). Laboratory evidence suggests the possibility of loss of midazolam at a higher temperature (37° C) which may be significant in combinations of midazolam and dexamethasone.[14]

Drug	Dose in syringe (mg)	Volume in syringe (ml)	Concentration (mg/ml)	Diluent	Outcome	Data Type
A	10		0.67			
B	1		0.07			
C	6.25	15	0.42	WFI	✓ (P) (24 h)	CLIN
D	40		2.67			
E	5		0.33			

Diamorphine (A), Glycopyrronium (B), Levomepromazine (C), Midazolam (D), and Octreotide (E)

Summary: No problems with physical stability encountered. To avoid irritation at the site of infusion, levomepromazine may be given as a subcutaneous bolus injection at doses below 50 mg (= 2 ml).

Drug	Dose in syringe (mg)	Volume in syringe (ml)	Concentration (mg/ml)	Diluent	Outcome	Data Type
A	30		1.25			
B	2.4		0.10			
C	50	24	2.08	WFI	✓ (P) (24 h)	CLIN
D	20		0.83			
E	0.6		0.03			
A	70		4.38			
B	1.2		0.08			
C	62.5	16	3.91	WFI	✓ (P) (24 h)	CLIN
D	10		0.63			
E	0.6		0.04			

Diamorphine (A), Glycopyrronium (B), Levomepromazine (C), Octreotide (D), and Ondansetron (E)

Summary: No problems with physical stability encountered. To avoid irritation at the site of infusion, levomepromazine may be given as a subcutaneous bolus injection at doses below 50 mg (= 2 ml).

Drug	Dose in syringe (mg)	Volume in syringe (ml)	Concentration (mg/ml)	Diluent	Outcome	Data Type
A	45**		1.88			
B	0.8		0.03			
C	18.75	24	0.78	NaCl	✓ (P) (24 h)	CLIN
D	0.6		0.03			
E	32		1.33			

**Diamorphine reconstituted with glycopyrronium.

Diamorphine (A), Glycopyrronium (B), Midazolam (C), Octreotide (D), and Ondansetron (E)

Summary: No problems with physical stability encountered.

Drug	Dose in syringe (mg)	Volume in syringe (ml)	Concentration (mg/ml)	Diluent	Outcome	Data Type
A	20**		3.33			
B	0.6		0.10			
C	5	12	0.83	NaCl	✓ (P) (12 h)	CLIN
D	0.15		0.03			
E	8		1.33			

**Diamorphine reconstituted with glycopyrronium.

Diamorphine (A), Haloperidol (B), Hyoscine Hydrobromide (C), Levomepromazine (D), and Midazolam (E)

Summary: No problems with physical stability encountered. Haloperidol was given in this case to control hiccups; generally haloperidol and levomepromazine should not be used together. To reduce irritation at the site of infusion, levomepromazine may also be given as a subcutaneous injection at doses below 50 mg (= 2 ml).

Drug	Dose in syringe (mg)	Volume in syringe (ml)	Concentration (mg/ml)	Diluent	Outcome	Data Type
A	30		1.76			
B	10		0.59			
C	1.2	17	0.07	WFI	✓ (P) (24 h)	CLIN
D	12.5		0.74			
E	40		2.35			

Diamorphine (A), Hyoscine Butylbromide (B), Levomepromazine (C), Midazolam (D), and Octreotide (E)

Summary: No problems with physical stability encountered. To avoid irritation at the site of infusion, levomepromazine may be given as a subcutaneous bolus injection at doses below 50 mg (= 2 ml).

Drug	Dose in syringe (mg)	Volume in syringe (ml)	Concentration (mg/ml)	Diluent	Outcome	Data Type
A	160		9.41			
B	120		7.06			
C	50	17	2.94	WFI	✓ (P) (24 h)	CLIN
D	15		0.88			
E	0.6		0.04			

Diamorphine (A), Hyoscine Butylbromide (B), Levomepromazine (C), Octreotide (D), and Ondansetron (E)

Summary: No problems with physical stability encountered. To avoid irritation at the site of infusion, levomepromazine may be given as a subcutaneous bolus injection at doses below 50 mg (= 2 ml).

Drug	Dose in syringe (mg)	Volume in syringe (ml)	Concentration (mg/ml)	Diluent	Outcome	Data Type
A	60**		2.73			
B	120		5.45			
C	18.75	22	0.85	NaCl	✓ (P) (24 h)	CLIN
D	0.6		0.03			
E	24		1.09			

**Reconstituted with hyoscine butylbromide.

Diamorphine (A), Hyoscine Butylbromide (B), Midazolam (C), Octreotide (D), and Ondansetron (E)

Summary: No problems with physical stability encountered.

Drug	Dose in syringe (mg)	Volume in syringe (ml)	Concentration (mg/ml)	Diluent	Outcome	Data Type
A	60**		3.33			
B	160		8.89			
C	5	18	0.28	–	✓ (P) (12 h)	CLIN
D	0.3		0.02			
E	12		0.67			

**Reconstituted with hyoscine butylbromide.

Morphine Hydrochloride (A), Dexamethasone (B), Haloperidol (C), Hyoscine Butylbromide (D), and Midazolam (E)

Summary: Physically incompatible at these concentrations. Dexamethasone is usually given as a subcutaneous bolus injection (depending upon volume of injection) or via a separate CSCI. However, if dexamethasone is to be mixed with other drugs, it should be the last constituent added to the maximally diluted syringe. There may be initial transient turbidity upon the addition of dexamethasone. Laboratory study suggests possibility of loss of midazolam at higher temperature (37° C) which may be significant in combinations of midazolam and dexamethasone.[14]

Drug	Dose in syringe (mg)	Volume in syringe (ml)	Concentration (mg/ml)	Diluent	Outcome	Data Type
A	420		1.68			
B	112		0.45			
C	52.5	250	0.21	NaCl	✗†	LAB[11]
D	420		1.68			
E	105		0.42			

†Infusion rate set at 1.5 ml/hour over the 7 days.

Tramadol (A), Dexamethasone (B), Haloperidol (C), Hyoscine Butylbromide (D), and Midazolam (E)

Summary: Physically incompatible at these concentrations. Dexamethasone is usually given as a subcutaneous bolus injection (depending upon volume of injection) or via a separate CSCI. However, if dexamethasone is to be mixed with other drugs, it should be the last constituent added to the maximally diluted syringe. There may be initial transient turbidity upon the addition of dexamethasone. Laboratory study suggests possibility of loss of midazolam at higher temperature (37° C) which may be significant in combinations of midazolam and dexamethasone.[14]

Drug	Dose in syringe (mg)	Volume in syringe (ml)	Concentration (mg/ml)	Diluent	Outcome	Data Type
A	2800		11.20			
B	112		0.45			
C	52.5	250	0.21	NaCl	✗[†]	LAB[11]
D	420		1.68			
E	105		0.42			

[†]Infusion rate set at 1.5 ml/hour over the 7 days.

References

1. Schneider J. (Personal communication-publication in preparation); 2004.

2. Stewart J,Warren F, King D,Venkateshwaran G, Fox J. (1998). Stability of ondansetron hydrochloride and 12 medications in plastic syringes. *Am J Health-Syst Pharm;* **55**:2630–2634.

3. Allwood MC. The stability of diamorphine alone and in combination with antiemetics in plastic syringes. *Palliat Med* 1991; **5**:330–333

4. Grassby PF, Hutchings L. Drug Combinations in syringe drivers: the compatibility and stability of diamorphine with cyclizine and haloperidol. *Palliat Med* 1997; **11**:217–224

5. Regnard C, Pashley S,Westrope F. Antiemetic/diamorphine mixture compatibility in infusion pumps. *Br J Pharm Prac* 1986; **8**:218–220

6. Myers KG, Trotman IF. Use of ketorolac by continuous subcutaneous infusion for the control of cancer-related pain. *Postgrad Med J.* 1994 May; **70**(823):359–62.

7. Fielding H, Kyaterekera N, Skellern GG, Tettey JN et al. The compatibility of octreotide acetate in the presence of diamorphine hydrochloride in polypropylene syringes. *Palliat Med* 2000; **14**:205–207.

8. Chandler SW, Trissel LA,Weinstein SM. Combined administration of opioids with selected drugs to manage pain and other cancer symptoms: initial safety screening for compatibility. *J Pain Symptom Manage* 1996; **12**:168–171.

9. Wilson K, Schneider J, Ravenscroft P. Stability of Midazolam and Fentanyl in Infusion Solutions. *J Pain Symptom Manage* 1998; **16**:52–58.

10. Walker SE, Iazzetta J, De Angelis C, Lau DCW. Stability and compatibility of combinations of hydromorphone and dimenhydrinate, lorazepam or prochlorperazine. *Can J Hosp Pharm* 1993; **46**:61–65.

11. Negro S, Luz Azuara M, Sanchez Y, Reyes R, Barcia E. Physical compatibility and in vivo evaluation of drug mixtures for subcutaneous infusion to cancer patients in palliative care. *Support Care Cancer* 2002; **10**:65–70.

12. Dickman A, Hunter S. Compatibility of oxycodone with palliative care supportive drugs. (Paper in preparation) 2004.

13. Gardiner PR. Compatibility of an injectable oxycodone formulation with typical diluents, syringes, tubings, infusion bags and drugs for potential co-administration. *Hospital Pharmacist* 2003; **10**:354–361.

14. Good P, Schneider J, Ravenscroft P. The compatibility and stability of midazolam and dexamethasone in infusion solutions. *J Pain Symptom Manage* 2004; **27**:471–475.

15. Ingallinera TS, Kapadia AJ, Hagman D, Klioze O. Compatibility of glycopyrrolate injection commonly used infusion solutions and additives. *Am J Hosp Pharm* 1979; **36**(4):508–510.

16. Barcia E, Reyes R, Luz Azuara M, Sanchez Y, Negro S. Compatibility of haloperidol and hyoscine-N-butylbromide in mixtures for subcutaneous infusion to cancer patients in palliative care. *Support Care Cancer* 2003; **11**:107–113.

17. Parker WA. Physical compatibility of ranitidine HCl with pre-operative injectable medications. *Can J Hosp Pharm* 1985; **38**:160–161.

18. Bradshaw K. Therapeutic Goods Administration Laboratory (Commonwealth Dept. of Health, Australia) Report (TGAL No: 9408/01081) 1990.

19. Schneider J, Good P and Ravenscroft PJ. Personal communication (publication in print); 2004.

Appendix 1

CSCI Administration Chart

Name:.............................	**Syringe Driver Nursing**
Unit no:............................	**Administration Record**
DOB:	
SD no:..............................	
Date commenced:.................	

All syringe drivers should be checked 4 hourly to ensure correct delivery, site viability and to check for signs of crystallization or precipitation. Nurses should sign and date when the driver is commenced and each time it is checked. Any problems should be recorded in the comments box. Inform the pharmacist or doctor should problems arise.

	Date	Dose(s)	Time	Volume in syringe (ml)	Site	Battery	Comments	Sign
Start Time		A)						
Start Volume		B)						
Duration ☐ 12hrs ☐ 24hrs		C) D)						
Start Time		A)						
Start Volume		B)						
Duration ☐ 12 hrs ☐ 24 hrs		C) D)						
Start Time		A)						
Start Volume		B)						
Duration ☐ 12 hrs ☐ 24 hrs		C) D)						
Start Time		A)						
Start Volume		B)						
Duration ☐ 12 hrs ☐ 24 hrs		C) D)						
Start Time		A)						
Start Volume		B)						
Duration ☐ 12 hrs ☐ 24 hrs		C) D)						

SAS Scheme

Special Access Scheme (SAS) Australia

The Special Access Scheme is an arrangement which provides a mechanism for the importing and/or supply of an unapproved therapeutic good for a patient. This is on a case by case basis. There are two categories for patients, with palliative care patients usually coming under Category A ('persons who are seriously ill with a condition from which death is reasonably likely to occur within a matter of months or from which premature death is reasonably likely to occur in the absence of early treatment').

In this case, patients, in consultation with their medical practitioner can obtain any therapeutic goods except those listed in Schedule 9 of the Standard for the Uniform Scheduling of Drugs and Poisons. For Category A patients, there is no need to gain prior approval from the Therapeutic Goods Administration (TGA). The medical practitioner must complete an 'Authority to Supply' form on which it is certified that:

- the patient is category A,
- informed consent has been obtained and
- the drug will be prescribed in accordance with good medical practice.

A copy of this form must be sent to the TGA within 4 weeks of the date of signing. A copy of this form is also sent to the sponsor of the product which provides them with the legal authority to supply the product.

This information was obtained from: http://www.tga.gov.au/docs/html/unapp.htm (Accessed May 2004).

Index